Clinician's Manual On Autism Spectrum Disorder

Editors
Evdokia Anagnostou
Jessica Brian

Clinician's Manual On Autism Spectrum Disorder

Adis

Editors
Evdokia Anagnostou and Jessica Brian
Autism Research Centre
Holland Bloorview Kids Rehabilitation Hospital
University of Toronto
Toronto, Ontario
Canada

ISBN 978-3-319-03055-5 ISBN 978-2-319-03056-2 (eBook)
DOI 10.1007/978-3-319-03056-2
Springer Cham Heidelberg New York Dordrecht London

Printed on acid-free paper

Adis is a brand of Springer
Springer is part of Springer Science+Business Media (www.springer.com)

Project editor: Katrina Dorn

Contents

Contributors

Stephanie Ameis
Susan Bryson
Daniel Coury
Christopher Kilmer
David Nicholas
Melanie Penner
Wendy Roberts
Sharon Smile
Isabel Smith
Peter Szatmari
Jennifer Walton
Lonnie Zwaigenbaum

Acknowledgments

We acknowledge the contribution of Dr Alana Iaboni at the Autism Research Centre, Bloorview Research Institute, University of Toronto, for her assistance with this manuscript.

Author biographies

Stephanie Ameis, MD, is the inaugural O'Brien Scholar and a clinician-scientist within the Child and Youth Mental Health Collaborative between the Centre for Addiction and Mental Health (CAMH), The Hospital for Sick Children and University of Toronto, Canada. She is Assistant Professor in the Department of Psychiatry, Faculty of Medicine at the University of Toronto. Dr. Ameis's clinical work focuses on providing assessment and care to children and youth with autism spectrum disorder (ASD) at CAMH. Her research work focuses on using advanced neuroimaging techniques to study how variation in the structure and function of brain circuits increases susceptibility for neuropsychiatric disorders that affect children and adolescents, with a focus on ASD, obsessive compulsive disorder (OCD), and disruptive behavior disorders. Dr. Ameis' research work also uses longitudinal brain imaging to track the effects of novel and existing treatments on brain structure and function over time.

Evdokia Anagnostou, MD, Senior Clinician Scientist, Bloorview Research Institute; Associate Professor, Department of Pediatrics, University of Toronto; Tier II Canada Research Chair in translational therapeutics in ASD. Dr. Evdokia Anagnostou is a child neurologist and a senior clinician scientist at the Bloorview Research Institute at the University of Toronto, Canada. She received her undergraduate degree from McGill University, completed her neurology training at McGill University in 2003, and a postdoctoral fellowship in autism/developmental disabilities at Mount Sinai School of Medicine in 2005. With a mission of improving outcomes and quality of life for children with ASD and their families, Dr. Anagnostou joined the Bloorview Research Institute in 2008, where she built and co-leads the Autism Research Centre. She has extensive funding in translational neuroscience and neuropsychopharmacology.

Jessica Brian, PhD, C.Psych, is a Psychologist and Clinician-Investigator at Holland Bloorview Kids Rehabilitation Hospital and Assistant Professor in the Department of Pediatrics at the University of Toronto, Canada. She received her PhD in Clinical-Developmental Psychology at York University in Toronto. Dr. Brian currently co-leads the Autism Research Centre at the Bloorview Research Institute with Dr. Evdokia Anagnostou. Her primary research interests include the emergence of ASD in infancy and toddlerhood, and the development, evaluation, and dissemination of evidence-based early intervention. She has been involved in a range of multi-site research programs aimed at understanding the emergence of ASD, characterizing its behavioral phenotype, and identifying genetic markers of ASD and related disorders. She is currently focusing on the development and evaluation of behavioural interventions for toddlers at risk for ASD. For over a decade, Dr. Brian has been involved in the Canadian Infant Siblings Study, now part of the international Autism Speaks Baby Sibs Research Consortium.

Susan Bryson, PhD, has been at Dalhousie University and the IWK since 2001 as Professor in Pediatrics and Psychology and first holder of the Craig Chair in Autism Research. Her research focuses on the early detection and treatment of ASD, as well as attention, emotion and temperament in ASD. In 2005, Dr. Bryson took the lead in establishing Nova Scotia's innovative Early Intensive Behavioral Intervention (EIBI) program for preschoolers with ASD. Building on the success of this program, she has since led the development of the Social ABCs, a parent-mediated intervention for toddlers with ASD. Dr. Bryson completed her PhD in Clinical Psychology at McGill University, Canada. She has received many prestigious awards, including both the Queen's Golden and Diamond Jubilee Medals for her contributions to autism.

Daniel Coury, MD, FAAP, is Professor of Pediatrics and Psychiatry in the College of Medicine at The Ohio State University and chief of the Section of Developmental and Behavioral Pediatrics at Nationwide Children's

Hospital in Columbus, Ohio. He conducts research and provides care for individuals with autism. His primary focus is his role as Medical Director for the Autism Speaks Autism Treatment Network, a network of hospitals and physicians dedicated to developing a model of comprehensive medical care for children and adolescents with autism.

Chris Kilmer, BSW, RSW, is a Research Coordinator in the Faculty of Social Work, University of Calgary (Edmonton Division) and the Department of Pediatrics at the University of Alberta, Canada. He brings experience in systematic and synthesis reviews in ASD, as well as qualitative methods analysis.

David Nicholas, PhD, RSW, Associate Professor in the Faculty of Social Work, University of Calgary (Edmonton Division); and is cross-appointed to the Department of Pediatrics at the University of Alberta, and the Research Insitute, The Hospital for Sick Children in Toronto. His area of research addresses quality of life, family support, and parenting with a focus on autism. He is currently involved in national and international studies addressing the impact of autism on families both at the point of diagnosis and over the course of child and adult development.

Melanie Penner, MD, FRCPC, is a developmental pediatrician with an interest in health service delivery for children with ASD. She completed her Bachelor of Health Sciences at McMaster University and Medical degree at Queen's University, Canada. She completed her residency in pediatrics and subspecialty residency in developmental pediatrics at the University of Toronto. Dr. Penner is currently pursuing a Master's degree in Health Services Research at the Institute of Health Policy in the Management and Evaluation through the Clinician Investigator program at the University of Toronto. Her research interest is health technology assessment of diagnostic methods and novel service delivery models for children with ASD.

Wendy Roberts, MD, is a developmental pediatrician who is now a Professor Emerita at the University of Toronto. She continues to be involved in autism care and advocacy in the community. She is Vice-Chair for the Clinical Expert Committee of the Ontario Ministry of Children and Youth, she collaborates in ongoing research in the genetics of autism and early identification and intervention, and is the Clinical Director of ISAND (Integrated Services for Autism and Neurodevelopmental Disorders), a Not-for-Profit Centre for Autism Care across the lifespan. Dr Roberts' research interests have focused on autism, its genetic etiology, its earliest signs, its developmental trajectory and diagnostic stability, associated syndromes which have autistic features (including epilepsy), and early developmentally appropriate intervention. She has been site Principal Investigator for several grants while co-directing the Autism Research Unit at the Hospital for Sick Children. In 2008, Dr Roberts successfully established Toronto as the first Canadian site of the Autism Treatment Network (ATN), a clinical database for autism on which numerous research studies have been built. She is also focused on helping to build a network of integrated services and continuum of care for individuals with ASD and their families from all over Ontario.

Sharon Smile, MD, completed her pediatric training at the University of The West Indies, Jamaica and a clinical fellowship in developmental pediatrics at The University of Toronto. She completed a Masters degree in clinical epidemiology at University of Toronto. Dr Smile is currently an Assistant Professor in the Department of Pediatrics, faculty of Medicine at the University of Toronto, and a developmental pediatrician at Holland Bloorview Kids Rehabilitation Hospital. Her interests include medical and mental health comorbidities seen among children diagnosed with ASD and intervention therapies to address comorbidities.

Isabel Smith, PhD, ScM, holds the Joan and Jack Craig Chair in Autism Research, and is a Professor in the Departments of Pediatrics, Psychology,

Neuroscience at Dalhousie University, based at the IWK Health Centre in Halifax, Nova Scotia, Canada. Dr. Smith's work as a clinical psychologist has focused on the promotion and implementation of evidence-based practices for early identification, diagnosis, and treatment of ASD. She has led studies of the impact of Nova Scotia's unique model of early intensive behavioral intervention for preschoolers with ASD since the program's inception in 2005. She is currently the principal investigator of a study comparing the cost-effectiveness of different early intervention models; other research interests include longitudinal studies of children and youth with ASD and treatment studies addressing behavioral disorders associated with ASD, such as anxiety and insomnia. As a faculty member of the Canadian Institutes of Health Research-funded Autism Research Training program, she contributes to the education of the next generation of ASD researchers.

Peter Szatmari, MD, is Chief of the Child and Youth Mental Health Collaborative between the Centre for Addiction and Mental Health (CAMH), the Hospital for Sick Children and the University of Toronto. Additionally, Dr. Szatmari holds the Patsy and Jamie Anderson Chair in Child and Youth Mental Health. Dr. Szatmari's investigative interests fall broadly into areas of psychiatric and genetic epidemiology, specifically: longitudinal studies of children with ASD and the factors associated with good outcomes; and the genetic etiology of autism including studying families with rare copy number variants and studies of infant siblings. Another area of interest is the developmental course of child and adolescent psychopathology including depression, eating disorders, oppositional behaviors, and anxiety disorders, with a particular area of concern being measurement issues and sampling by family unit rather than by individuals.

Jennifer Walton, MD, MPH, FAAP, is Assistant Professor of Pediatrics in the College of Medicine at The Ohio State University, and an attending physician in the Section of Developmental and Behavioral Pediatrics at Nationwide Children's Hospital in Columbus, Ohio. She provides care for individuals with ASD, ADHD, and other developmental disabilities. Her primary focus is her role is as Medical Director for the Williams Syndrome Clinic, medical lead of the Southeastern Ohio Interdisciplinary Assessment Team, and coordinator of the pediatric resident and medical student clinical training for developmental and behavioral pediatrics at Nationwide Children's Hospital.

Lonnie Zwaigenbaum, MD, PhD, completed his pediatric training at Queen's University, and his clinical fellowship in developmental pediatrics at The Hospital for Sick Children in Toronto, Canada. He completed a research fellowship and Masters degree in health research methodology at McMaster University. Dr. Zwaigenbaum's research focuses on early behavioral and biological markers and developmental trajectories in children and youth with ASD. He currently holds an Alberta Innovates Health Solutions Health Scholar Award and the Stollery Children's Hospital Foundation Chair in Autism Research. Dr. Zwaigenbaum is a Professor in the Department of Pediatrics at the University of Alberta, and the co-director of the Autism Research Centre based at the Glenrose Rehabilitation Hospital.

Chapter 1

Introduction

Evdokia Anagnostou, Jessica Brian

Autism spectrum disorder (ASD) has been redefined in the most recent Diagnostic and Statistical Manual of Mental Disorders (DSM-5) to include deficits in social communication and repetitive behaviors/restricted interests [1]. Language and cognitive deficits are now considered orthogonal to the diagnosis. A series of specifiers are available to allow for better description of each individual child and a severity matrix has been proposed for the first time. However, the most significant implication of the DSM-5 changes is that clinicians are challenged to admit that they do not yet know how to describe the heterogeneity of the spectrum in terms of biologically distinct groups.

There has been an explosion in genomics and systems neuroscience relating to ASD, which has the potential to start bringing clarity to the field. For example, at least 10% of children with ASD have copy-number variants (CNV), which are believed to be associated with their disorder [2]; early whole genome sequencing would suggest that up to 50% of children have de novo and rare inherited mutations related to their phenotype [3]. Several of these findings are already being developed into diagnostic tests. Of particular interest, however, is that despite the very high number of genomic variations seen in ASD and related disorders, network analyses would suggest that such variation maps on to distinct biological processes, including synaptic function, chromatin remodelling, and transcription regulation, among others. Some of these pathways are

E. Anagnostou and J. Brian (eds.), *Clinician's Manual on Autism Spectrum Disorder*, DOI 10.1007/978-3-319-03056-2_1

informing our approach to treatment development so that, for the first time, it seems reasonable to expect that treatments may be developed through the translational route.

Much debate exists around the increasing prevalence of the disorder, with recent Centers for Disease Control and Prevention (CDC) numbers estimating that 1 in 68 children in the US has ASD [4]. Whether this represents reclassification or whether there are environment-by-gene interactions responsible for true new cases remains to be established, the fact remains that higher numbers of children are accessing our health care systems. This, in turn, requires a systems approach to developing evidence-based guidelines for the screening, diagnosis, and treatment of ASD across the lifespan.

In addition, the increased prevalence of the multitude of co-occurring conditions (both psychiatric and medical) in this population increases the burden to both mental and physical health systems. Whether such co-occurring conditions reveal something about the biological heterogeneity of ASD or whether their presence may predict specific biological phenotypes remains to be seen. However, their presence interacts with core symptom domain deficits to significantly affect long-term outcomes and quality of life. As such, prompt detection of such conditions and treatment may be as critical to the long-term functional outcomes of people with ASD, as is early detection and treatment of core symptom domains.

In this book, the authors, who are experts in their respective fields, review the evidence across several domains of interest to clinicians, including effective screening and diagnostic procedures, pharmacological, psychological, and educational treatments, and the impact of ASD on families. The evidence for early detection and behavioral intervention as predictors of optimal outcomes is strong and the authors summarize such evidence and provide concrete guidance to clinicians about best practices.

Although no medications have been approved for the treatment of core symptom domains of ASD, there is evidence to support their judicious use for the treatment of associated symptoms such as attention deficit hyperactivity disorder, anxiety, and irritability/aggression, among others. The evidence for such a practice is reviewed and recommendations are made. In addition, particular attention is paid to the characterization of psychiatric and medical co-occurring conditions and approaches to their management. Lastly, we recognize that the burden of ASD-related dysfunction is not only experienced by individuals with ASD themselves but also by their families and caregivers. Understanding the strengths and challenges of children, youth, and adults with ASD, as well as their families, is critical in order to support them proactively and within an evidence-based family-centered health care system.

The aim of this clinician's manual is to be an essential resource for clinicians caring for individuals with ASD. The field has made significant gains in our understanding of ASD and the factors that predict optimal outcomes and this book will serve to facilitate the implementation of evidence-based screening, diagnosis, and treatment of individuals on the autism spectrum.

References

1 American Psychiatric Association. *Diagnostic and Statistical Manual of Mental Disorders*. 5th Edition. Washington, DC: American Psychiatric Association; 2013.

2 Devlin B, Scherer SW. Genetic architecture in autism spectrum disorder, *Curr Opin Genet Dev*. 2012;22:229-237.

3 Jiang YH, Yuen RKC, Jin X, et al. Detection of clinically relevant genetic variants in autism spectrum disorder by whole-genome sequencing. *Am J Hum Genet*. 2013;2:249-263.

4 Centers for Disease Control and Prevention (CDC). Data and Statistics: Autism Spectrum Disorder (ASD). *CDC*. www.cdc.gov/ncbddd/autism/data.html. Accessed February 4, 2015.

Chapter 2

Diagnosis: screening, surveillance, assessment, and formulation

Melanie Penner, Lonnie Zwaigenbaum, Wendy Roberts

Key Learning Objectives

By the end of this chapter, readers will be able to:

- identify necessary team members and define team member roles for the diagnostic assessment of autism spectrum disorder (ASD);
- recognize how the caregiver history, history from other sources, physical examination, informal observation, and formal observation contribute to the diagnostic assessment;
- conceptualize and integrate the assessment findings into a formulation that addresses the diagnostic question in the context of the child's neurodevelopmental profile; and
- communicate the findings of the assessment effectively with families, providing an informative summary and interpretation.

Assessment of autism spectrum disorder: surveillance and screening

Community health care providers and other professionals involved in supporting optimal child development (eg, early childhood educators) play a critical role in working with parents to identify early signs of ASD. Screening and surveillance are complementary processes aimed at identifying children who require further assessment, with an overall goal of reducing or preventing subsequent disability through earlier initiation of

E. Anagnostou and J. Brian (eds.), *Clinician's Manual on Autism Spectrum Disorder*, DOI 10.1007/978-3-319-03056-2_2

intervention [1]. Screening refers to administering and scoring a specific instrument (eg, parent questionnaire) to identify at-risk individuals in need of further assessment. 'First stage' (or universal) screening targets all children regardless of level of concern or other risk factors; 'second stage' screening is limited to children who are flagged due to identified concerns, a positive family history, or other risk factors (eg, medical diagnosis with a known association with ASD).

In contrast, surveillance consists of an ongoing process that includes inquiry about parents' concerns and observations of the child, generally in the context of an ongoing clinical relationship (ie, by a community physician), to obtain an overall picture of the child's developmental health over time [2]. In that context, decisions about referral for further evaluation are made based on clinical judgment. Developmental surveillance can include the administration of standardized tools (including screening questionnaires), but with the aim of obtaining additional information to help inform clinical decision-making, rather than using scoring cut-points as a basis for referral.

There is growing evidence supporting the clinical utility of ASD screening by community health providers (ie, predictive value of a positive screen, potential to detect children earlier than by general monitoring of developmental concerns) [3–5]. However, most screening research focuses on accuracy (ie, 'correct' classification of children with ASD, but not children who do not have ASD, as being at-risk and in need of further assessment based on a positive screen) rather than meaningful end-points such as age of diagnosis, access to early intervention and long-term outcomes [6]. As a result, there is still considerable debate as to what should currently be considered 'best practice', with some authors advocating for broad-scale implementation of universal ASD screening as early as 18 months in accordance with current American Academy of Pediatrics recommendations [7,8], while others continue to argue that more evidence is needed [9,10].

There also remains uncertainty about the relative merits of a first- or second-stage screening strategy for ASD. First-stage screening has the potential advantage of higher sensitivity (and thus, more children with

ASD being correctly identified at an early age), but also tends to identify more children who do not have ASD (ie, false positives), with potential implications for parental stress and straining service capacity for appropriate follow-up assessments. Second-stage screening also presents challenges. To be effective, general developmental surveillance must correctly identify children with ASD for further assessment; however, there is evidence that current screening methods may miss some children who would otherwise be flagged by ASD-specific screens [5,11].

Recent research advances help reconcile the advantages and disadvantages of first- versus second-stage screening by offering a combined, integrated approach, while at the same time, further supporting the overall utility of ASD screening. For example, the Modified-Checklist for Autism in Toddlers (M-CHAT) is an ASD screening tool which has been evaluated in large community samples of 16- to 30-month-olds assessed during well child visits. By combining a 23-item parent questionnaire with a structured follow-up interview to clarify items endorsed by parents, the M-CHAT essentially functions as a combined level 1 and level 2 screening tool, with approximately 50–60% of screen positive children who are referred and assessed being subsequently diagnosed with ASD [12–14]. Recently, Robins et al [15] reported validation data for a new version of this instrument, the 'Modified Checklist for Autism in Toddlers, Revised with Follow-up' (M-CHAT-R/F). The questionnaire was reduced to 20 items and a scoring algorithm with three risk ranges was developed. Children in the 'low-risk' range (<3 items endorsed) did not require the follow-up interview or any other additional evaluation (93% of all cases). Children in the 'medium-risk' range (3–7 items endorsed; 6% of all cases) required the follow-up interview to clarify their risk for ASD; if at least 2 items remained positive, then referral for diagnostic evaluation was indicated. Children in the 'high-risk' range (8 or more items endorsed; 1% of all cases) were at sufficiently high risk to be referred directly for diagnostic assessment without the follow-up interview. This revised scoring and referral algorithm reduced the initial screen positive rate (from 9.2–7.2%) and increased the overall rate of ASD detection (67 vs. 45 per 10,000) [15].

Wetherby et al [16] have adopted a similar strategy with the Communication and Symbolic Behavioral Scales Infant Toddler Checklist (CSBS-ITC), recommending that children identified by this broadband screener, designed to detect communication delays, have an additional assessment for behavioral 'red flags' [17] to further determine which children require an ASD diagnostic assessment. The ITC has been demonstrated to have very high sensitivity in a community sample, detecting over 90% of children with ASD by age 24 months [16], although evaluation of the care pathway that includes the second level behavioral assessment has not yet been reported.

As ASD screening in community settings continues to be evaluated [6] and health policy regarding screening continues to evolve, developmental specialists will continue to have an important role in working with their community colleagues to encourage careful monitoring for early signs of ASD, understanding of referral and care pathways, and working collaboratively with families though the assessment process. This collaboration extends to helping parents understand the diagnosis and to navigate the service system so that the child and family access appropriate supports and services in a timely way. Establishing a positive working relationship with community health professionals also lays the foundation for ongoing co-management of the child in relation to their diagnosis, and other potential physical and emotional health issues that may arise [18].

Team structure and function

The success of a diagnostic assessment hinges on effective teamwork. This is true whether the diagnosis is made with a multidisciplinary team of health care providers in a tertiary care setting or a single clinician in a community practice. Clinicians learn to appreciate that they work in concert with the child and his or her family to gather and synthesize information that may lead to a diagnosis but will, more importantly, foster a greater understanding of the child's neurodevelopmental profile. This profile informs not only the family, but also service providers and members of the family's community support system.

Most jurisdictions do not mandate which professionals need to be involved in the diagnostic assessment. Each child will present with unique challenges, and different team members may need to be consulted with each new case. Table 2.1 lists potential contributions by family members and professionals.

Because of high demand for ASD assessments, constrained health care resources and limited geographic access to tertiary care centers, an in-person multidisciplinary team assessment may not be possible. In such cases, clinicians may be part of a 'virtual' team, in which assessments occurring across time and locations are incorporated into the diagnostic formulation. While virtual teams may allow for some efficiency, they create an additional challenge for the team leader to synthesize information from various contexts. Technological advances can now be used to

Team member	Role
Leader	Coordinates elements of the assessment
	Responsible for communication of assessment results to family
	Develops management and follow-up plan
Caregivers	Provide bulk of history
	Provide consent to contact other individuals with knowledge of child
Siblings	Source of valuable information
	Provide clinicians an opportunity to observe peer interaction
Physician	Medical and developmental history (+/– standardized interview tools)
	Physical examination
	Observation (formal and informal)
	Coordination of further testing (biochemical, genetic, imaging, etc)
Psychologist	Developmental history (+/– standardized interview)
	Observation (formal and informal)
	Intelligence or developmental assessment tools
	Other formal neuropsychological tests (adaptive function, executive function, achievement, attention/hyperactivity/ impulsivity)
Speech-language pathologist	Formal assessment of language and communication skills
	Assessment of speech and language pragmatics
Occupational therapist	Sensory profile
	Motor coordination

Table 2.1 Team members and potential contributions to diagnostic assessment.

connect team members across settings to allow valuable team discussions to occur with all members present, which often provides richer insight into the child's profile.

Components of diagnostic assessment

Patient history

A thorough and accurate history provides the foundation for a diagnosis of ASD. Because it is often the first part of the assessment, it also allows the clinician to develop a therapeutic interaction with caregivers. This rapport greatly influences the tone of the assessment and can improve receptiveness to the results of the evaluation.

The clinician should begin by asking about the caregivers' understanding of the reason for the referral and their goals for the assessment. Caregivers may or may not have been told about the possibility of ASD. To provide informed consent for the assessment, caregivers must know that you will be evaluating for ASD. Some approaches to broach this topic include:

> *"Sometimes families have specific things they want us to look for, such as autism spectrum disorder or attention deficit hyperactivity disorder. Is there anything you'd like us to look for in your child?"*

> *"We will be looking at all areas of your child's development; however, your doctor wrote that (child's name) has challenges with his/her (language/social skills/play). In these cases, it is important that we look for any signs of an autism spectrum disorder."*

It is also important to start the interaction by explaining the various components of the assessment, including the amount of time and number of appointments you anticipate. By helping caregivers understand what to expect, clinicians can foster a trusting environment that will relieve some anxiety for the family.

The clinician should then gather more information about the caregivers' concerns and observations that have been communicated to them by other people in the child's life. It is important to solicit information about how the child functions in multiple environments, such as daycare, school and recreational activities.

The history should explicitly cover all DSM diagnostic criteria with clear examples of each criterion when present. The Autism Diagnostic Interview – Revised (ADI-R) [19] is a standardized interview that can be completed by an experienced clinician in approximately 1.5 to 2 hours and is useful for children with a mental age of at least 2 years of age. The ADI-R consists of 93 items grouped into domains of Language/Communication; Reciprocal Social Interactions; and Restricted, Repetitive, and Stereotyped Behaviors and Interests.

The developmental history should cover all developmental domains regardless of the reason for referral. While the focus should be on current skills, the progression of communication and social skills is essential to elicit, as is any significant loss of previously acquired skills (regression). Many clinicians choose to incorporate a standardized adaptive skills interview, such as the Vineland Adaptive Behavior Scales II (VABS-II) [20], to measure current performance across domains of development. The VABS-II can be incorporated into a developmental history and provides a standardized measure of the child's current developmental function with standard scores, percentiles, and age equivalents.

The history should also include a thorough past medical history, including the pregnancy and neonatal period. The review of systems should pay particular attention to hearing, vision, sleep, nutrition, and gastrointestinal symptoms. A three-generation family history should be elicited including ASD, developmental delays, school failure, learning disabilities, language delays, attention deficit hyperactivity disorder, anxiety (particularly social anxiety) or other psychiatric conditions, hearing impairment, seizures, congenital anomalies, multiple spontaneous abortions, and consanguinity. A social history, including living situation, employment, and support is important and may influence the management plan.

Questionnaires

In cases where a formal ASD interview tool such as the ADI-R is not feasible, clinicians may choose to provide caregivers with questionnaires, which are less time-consuming and can be completed between appointments. These questionnaires can also be given to other individuals who have frequent contact with the child, such as child care staff and teachers.

The Social Communication Questionnaire (SCQ) [21] is a screening tool based on the ADI-R that can be used for children over 4 years with a mental age over 2 years of age. It consists of 40 'yes/no' items and can be quickly and easily completed by caregivers. Some clinicians prefer to use it as a guide in a semi-structured interview format to cover the diagnostic criteria systematically during the history taking.

The Social Responsiveness Scale-2 (SRS-2) [22] is designed to identify social impairment that is seen in ASD and to differentiate it from social difficulties that occur in other disorders. It can be completed for children as young as 30 months and takes approximately 15 minutes for caregivers to complete.

Informal observation

The child may not need to be present for the entire developmental history; however, it is important to observe the child in the same room as the caregivers for part of the assessment. This time is filled with rich information about the interaction between the child and caregivers, how the child adapts to the new environment, the child's attempts to obtain, maintain, and direct the caregiver's attention, and how the caregiver deals with undesirable behavior.

Formal observation

In most cases, clinicians will use a formal observational tool to help them systematically observe behaviors consistent with DSM criteria. The Autism Diagnostic Observation Schedule, 2nd edition (ADOS-2) [23] is a frequently utilized semi-structured interaction that provides structured opportunities to assess communication, social interaction, play, and restricted and repetitive behaviors. Clinicians must undergo training to administer and score the ADOS. Modules 1–4 provide cut-off scores for ASD and can be used in children as young as 31 months; the Toddler Module provides ranges of concern (instead of cut-off scores) and can be used in children between 12 and 30 months of age [23].

The Childhood Autism Rating Scale (CARS-2) is a brief observational scale with 15 items that can be used in children aged 2 and older.

Physical examination

A physical examination by a physician is a necessary component of the diagnostic assessment because of the many medical comorbidities associated with ASD (see Chapter 3). If a physician is not part of the diagnostic team, the child's pediatrician can perform a thorough examination after the diagnosis is made. The physical examination should be comprehensive, with particular attention to growth parameters and dysmorphic features. A thorough neurologic examination is warranted in all children with suspected ASD.

Because of sensory processing difficulties, children with ASD often have difficulty with the physical examination. It is best to attempt the exam when the child is comfortable with the environment and in a good mood. Because the diagnosis itself does not rely on the results of the physical examination, it may be appropriate to complete it at a later date.

Additional assessment components

Other types of assessments, as listed in Table 2.1, may be useful depending on the individual needs of the child. At a minimum, hearing and vision development must be documented prior to a diagnosis of ASD. A psycho-educational assessment can be performed at the time of diagnosis or when the child reaches school age. Many children will also benefit from speech and occupational therapy assessments, which may help to inform the diagnosis and formulation or can be part of the management plan.

Formulation and feedback

The formulation synthesizes the results of the assessment and feedback involves presenting diagnostic impressions. The formulation is typically a written summary of findings from the patient assessment(s) and is what will be consulted by family and service providers going forward after a diagnosis. Feedback involves presenting the formulation and sharing a diagnosis; parents have described the impact of the feedback session as "the hour changed our lives forever." Because of the importance of the feedback session, it is useful for the clinician to finalize a formulation before giving a diagnosis.

Formulation

Introducing the formulation section with a brief summary of patient information and observations collected from parents, the referring clinician, and others in the community sets the stage for making a diagnosis. It can include relevant developmental and medical history, symptoms that address the diagnostic criteria, and how initial concerns about ASD developed. After gathering a patient history, results of assessments can be briefly summarized, along with reports from teachers, childcare professionals, and other relevant individuals who have come into contact with the patient. This information can consist of both formal and informal observations relating to the criteria that led to a diagnostic impression.

One method of doing this is via a 'diagnostic paragraph' which may help a parent or caregiver to better understand the diagnostic criteria that appear to have been met. An explanation of the current severity, prognosis, and ASD subtype (even if an unofficial one, such as an Asperger's disorder) may be included in the diagnostic paragraph or may warrant a separate discussion. Similarly, the clinician should explain how ASD may affect dimensions of development, such as language, cognition, developmental status, and functional or adaptive skills. Other coexisting diagnoses such as intellectual disability, language impairment, motor speech disorders, attention deficit hyperactivity disorder, and social or other forms of anxiety disorders need to be discussed.

An itemized management plan and list of recommendations should accompany a diagnosis. This can include a medical follow-up and investigation, referrals to community services, access to helpful resources for families, and strategies tailored to the child's various environments to promote engagement and learning. This list should be as comprehensive as possible, as it is often referenced by families and health care professionals throughout the patient's life.

Feedback

A feedback session follows a similar structure to the formulation. At each stage, the clinician should ensure the parents/caregiver understands and agrees with clinical observations. This will help the family to appreciate the evidence upon which a diagnosis is based and help to prevent later disagreement or confusion.

Some clinicians find it hard to use the term 'autism' with parents and caregivers; this could be made less difficult if the medical terms have been discussed throughout the assessment process and are reiterated during the feedback session. After presenting the evidence, clinicians must communicate the diagnosis in a clear and unambiguous statement. An example of a way to communicate the diagnosis is as follows:

> *"[Child's name] has difficulty sharing his/her feelings with another person. He/she has very focused interests and insists that the world 'stays the same.' He/she also has intense sensory interests and repetitive movements. When we see this combination, the name we give it is autism spectrum disorder. Based on my assessment, he/she has autism spectrum disorder."*

Families will have varying reactions in the moments after they receive the diagnosis. Though the ensuing silence can be uncomfortable, it is important to let families reflect on the impact of the diagnosis. This is the time when the family may wish to guide the remainder of the feedback session with the many questions they may have about their child.

Prognosis will often be the first question from parents. Explaining the predictors of outcome, such as early identification and intervention, intellectual level, age when language emerges, and coexistence of other medical issues, can be helpful for parents. Unfortunately, there is still a great deal of uncertainty in predicting the outcome of individuals with ASD and this must also be communicated to the family. Discussion of a management plan is vital but may be difficult during the first session when the diagnosis is shared. The family may require a number of sessions to discuss the modality and intensity of interventions, medical issues, diet and nutrition, alternative and complementary therapies, and management of difficult behaviors and emotion dysregulation.

References

1 Zwaigenbaum L. Screening, risk and early identification of autism spectrum disorders. In: Amaral D, Dawson G, Geschwin D, eds. *Autism Spectrum Disorders*. New York: Oxford University Press; 2011:75-89.

2 Dworkin PH. British and American recommendations for developmental monitoring: the role of surveillance. *Pediatrics*. 1989;84:1000-1010.

3 Barton ML, Dumont-Mathieu T, Fein D. Screening young children for autism spectrum disorders in primary practice. *J Autism Dev Disord*. 2012;42:1165-1174.

4 Herlihy LE, Brooks B, Dumont-Mathieu T, et al. Standardized screening facilitates timely diagnosis of autism spectrum disorders in a diverse sample of low-risk toddlers. *J Dev Behav Pediatr*. 2014;35:85-92.

5 Wiggins LD, Piazza V, Robins DL. Comparison of a broad-based screen versus disorder-specific screen in detecting young children with an autism spectrum disorder. *Autism*. 2014;18:76-84.

6 Daniels AM, Halladay AK, Shih A, Elder LM, Dawson G. Approaches to enhancing the early detection of autism spectrum disorders: a systematic review of the literature. *J Am Acad Child Adolesc Psychiatry*. 2014;53:141-152.

7 Lipkin PH, Hyman SL. Should all children be screened for autism spectrum disorders? Yes: merging science, policy, and practice. *Am Fam Physician*. 2011;84:361-367.

8 Myers SM, Johnson CP, American Academy of Pediatrics Council on Children With Disabilities. Management of children with autism spectrum disorders. *Pediatrics*. 2007;120:1162-1182.

9 Al-Qabandi M, Gorter JW, Rosenbaum P. Early autism detection: are we ready for routine screening? *Pediatrics*. 2011;128:e211-e217.

10 Campos-Outcalt D. Should all children be screened for autism spectrum disorders? No: screening is not ready for prime time. *Am Fam Physician*. 2011;84:377-378.

11 Pinto-Martin JA, Young LM, Mandell DS, Poghosyan L, Giarelli E, Levy SE. Screening strategies for autism spectrum disorders in pediatric primary care. *J Dev Behav Pediatr*. 2008;29:345-350.

12 Chlebowski C, Robins DL, Barton ML, Fein D. Large-scale use of the modified checklist for autism in low-risk toddlers. *Pediatrics*. 2013;131:e1121-e1127.

13 Kleinman JM, Robins DL, Ventola PE, et al. The modified checklist for autism in toddlers: a follow-up study investigating the early detection of autism spectrum disorders. *J Autism Dev Disord*. 2008;38:827-839.

14 Robins DL. Screening for autism spectrum disorders in primary care settings. *Autism*. 2008;12:537-556.

15 Robins DL, Casagrande K, Barton M, Chen A, Dumont-Mathieu T, Fein D. Validation of the modified checklist for autism in toddlers, revised with follow-up (M-CHAT-R/F). *Pediatrics*. 2014;133:37-45.

16 Wetherby AM, Brosnan-Maddox S, Peace V, Newton L. Validation of the infant-toddler checklist as a broadband screener for autism spectrum disorders from 9 to 24 months of age. *Autism*. 2008;12:487-511.

17 Wetherby AM, Woods J, Allen L, Cleary J, Dickinson H, Lord C. Early indicators of autism spectrum disorders in the second year of life. *J Autism Dev Disord*. 2004;34:473-493.

18 Anagnostou E, Zwaigenbaum L, Szatmari P, et al. Autism spectrum disorder: advances in evidence-based practice. *CMAJ*. 2014;186:509-519.

19 Rutter M, Lecouteur A, Lord C. *Autism Diagnostic Interview- Revised (ADI-R)*. Torrance, CA: WPS; 2003. www.wpspublish.com. Accessed February 4, 2015.

20 Sparrow S, Cicchetti D, Balla D. *Vineland adaptive behavior scales, second edition.* San Antonio, TX: Pearson; 2005. www.pearsonclinical.com. Accessed January 4, 2015.

21 Rutter M, Baily A, Lord C. *Social Communication Questionnaire (SCQ).* Torrance, CA: WPS; 2003. www.wpspublish.com. Accessed January 4, 2015.

22 Constantino J. *Social Responsiveness Scale (SRS-2).* Second edition. Torrance, CA: WPS; 2012. www.wpspublish.com. Accessed January 4, 2015.

23 Lord C, Rutter M, Dilavore P, Risi S, Gotham K, Bishop S. *Autism Diagnostic Observation Schedule.* Second edition. Torrance, CA: WPS; 2012. www.wpspublish.com. Accessed February 4, 2015.

Chapter 3

Common psychiatric comorbidities and their assessment

Stephanie H Ameis, Peter Szatmari

Key Learning Objectives

By the end of this chapter, readers will be able to identify:

- recent evidence that indicates that a majority of children and adolescents with autism spectrum disorder (ASD) meet symptom criteria for at least one psychiatric disorder (particularly anxiety);
- DSM-5 guidance for diagnosing comorbid ASD and a psychiatric condition;
- limited range of validated tools available to help support clinicians in assessing for comorbid psychiatric disorders in ASD;
- necessity of clinical judgment in combination with direct observation, careful history taking with caregivers, and collateral information to determine whether a comorbid psychiatric diagnosis should be made in individuals with ASD;
- preliminary treatment studies that have demonstrated efficacy in treating other psychiatric symptoms (eg, attention deficit hyperactivity disorder [ADHD]) symptoms in individuals with ASD.

Introduction

Recent studies indicate that psychiatric comorbidity is common in ASD, that rates of problematic psychiatric symptoms are higher in ASD than

E. Anagnostou and J. Brian (eds.), *Clinician's Manual on Autism Spectrum Disorder*, DOI 10.1007/978-3-319-03056-2_3

in the general population, and that comorbid psychiatric disorders can significantly impair functioning and interfere with therapeutic and scholastic progress [1,2]. However, the identification and appropriate management of psychiatric comorbidity in ASD (and research in this area) was likely hindered by diagnostic restrictions set out in the previous edition of the Diagnostic and Statistical Manual of Mental Disorders (DSM-IV-TR), which precluded conferring a combined diagnosis of both ASD and certain psychiatric disorders, such as ADHD or social anxiety disorder (social phobia) [3]. Over the last decade, studies indicating that individuals with ASD struggle with high rates of psychiatric comorbidity have led to important changes in diagnostic criteria in the 2013 edition (DSM-5) that remove previous barriers to diagnosing comorbid psychiatric disorders in this population [4]. However, there are currently few tools to help clinicians conduct an assessment of psychiatric comorbidity in ASD. This chapter will summarize available evidence on the prevalence of psychiatric comorbidity in ASD, highlight relevant changes to the DSM-5, and provide general principles that can be applied in the clinical context to guide assessment and management of common comorbid psychiatric disorders in this population.

Prevalence of psychiatric comorbidity

Within the past decade, a number of research studies have been conducted using psychiatric assessment instruments to assess psychiatric comorbidity in ASD. Studies of children and adolescents with ASD (n=109–414) have indicated that roughly 70% of young people with ASD, recruited from the community, meet symptom criteria for at least one psychiatric disorder [5–7]. Strikingly, close to half of those with ASD and psychiatric comorbidity may meet criteria for more than one comorbid psychiatric disorder [6,7]. Rates of ADHD and anxiety disorders are consistently found to be high in studies of psychiatric comorbidity in ASD, with results indicating that these disorders may be present in approximately 40–50% of affected children and adolescents [6–10]. A recent meta-analysis including data from over 2000 children and adolescents indicated that among the anxiety disorders, specific phobia was most common in ASD (affecting 30%), followed by obsessive compulsive (OCD; 17%), social anxiety (16%), generalized anxiety (15%), separation anxiety (9%), and panic disorder (2%) [8]. While comorbid oppositional defiant disorder (ODD), enuresis/encopresis, sleep and mood disorders are also commonly reported in children and adolescents with ASD, prevalence rates for these disorders are more variable between studies [7,11]. Although problems with tantrums and aggression may not meet criteria for a specific psychiatric disorder, it is important to note that problems in these areas are common among children with ASD, regardless of age, ability, or schooling [12]. A small number of studies conducted in high functioning adults recruited from mental health clinics (n=54–122) have pointed to high rates of comorbid major depressive disorder in this population (53–70%), in addition to ADHD (43%) and anxiety disorders (50%) [13,14]. Limited data indicate that rates of psychiatric comorbidity and intellectual disability in adults with ASD may be similar to those seen in adults with intellectual disability without ASD [15]. Although some evidence has indicated that comorbid psychiatric disorders may be more common in higher functioning individuals with ASD [16], other studies have not found a clear relationship between psychiatric comorbidity and ASD severity, IQ, or adaptive functioning [7]. As very few studies have examined putative risk factors for psychiatric comorbidity in individuals with ASD, further work is needed in this area.

The DSM-5 and diagnosis of psychiatric comorbidity in autism spectrum disorder

The DSM-5 recognizes that individuals with ASD suffer from high rates of psychiatric comorbidity and includes significant changes to diagnostic criteria from the previous edition of the DSM that facilitate diagnosis of comorbid disorders in this population [4]. The previous edition (DSM-IV-TR) did not address comorbid psychiatric disorders as part of the diagnostic criteria for pervasive developmental disorders (PDD) (encompassing diagnoses of autistic disorder, Asperger's disorder, and pervasive developmental disorder-not otherwise specified) [3]. Furthermore, ADHD could not be diagnosed if symptoms occurred exclusively during the course of PDD, and social phobia could only be diagnosed in children with the capacity to form age-appropriate social relationships [3]. In sharp contrast, the DSM-5 now includes a separate specifier within the diagnostic criteria for ASD that enables clinicians to indicate whether ASD is "associated with another neurodevelopmental, mental, or behavioral disorder" in their patients [4]. The DSM-5 text also clearly states that when criteria for ASD and ADHD, anxiety, depressive or other comorbid disorders are met, both (or even multiple) diagnoses should be made, thereby removing previous barriers to diagnosing comorbid psychiatric disorders in this population.

Assessment of psychiatric comorbidity

Important considerations

A number of diagnostic challenges still face clinicians attempting to diagnose psychiatric comorbidity in ASD [17]. First, most standardized diagnostic interviews assessing psychiatric symptoms in young people have not been validated for ASD. Further, language impairments in ASD can lead to challenges in eliciting thoughts and feelings that are often used to make psychiatric diagnoses. Finally, the symptoms of ASD and comorbid disorders (and impairment caused by these symptoms) may overlap resulting in difficulty distinguishing between symptoms and secondary impairment that are part of the ASD presentation versus those that are part of the presentation for a comorbid psychiatric disorder [17], versus impairments that are compounded by both ASD symptoms and psychiatric comorbidity (eg, social impairment due to ASD and social anxiety disorder).

General principles of assessment

There are a number of helpful strategies that clinicians may use when assessing for the presence of psychiatric comorbidity in ASD. First, a comprehensive assessment of an individual with ASD should include both direct observation of the patient and a full history from the patient, parents/family, or other care providers around the presence of ASD/psychiatric/medical symptoms and secondary functional impairment [18]. Based on the extant literature, and in light of DSM-5 diagnostic criteria, clinicians providing care to individuals with ASD must carefully screen for all commonly comorbid psychiatric symptoms (ie, ADHD symptoms, anxiety, mood, sleep and elimination problems, and challenging behaviors) in this population. As individuals with ASD often present with more than one comorbid psychiatric disorder, it is important to assess for disorders that tend to co-occur (eg, anxiety and depressive disorders) both in the general population and in individuals with ASD [19]. Given the common occurrence of challenging (including aggressive) behaviors in ASD and the potential safety risk that self-injury and injury to others may cause [11], clinicians must inquire about the presence of these behaviors in their patients, and establish both triggers (eg, anxiety, pain, sensitivity to transitions) and the function of these behaviors (eg, escape, avoidance, attention) [20]. Evaluating antecedents, behaviors, and consequences ('ABCs') of challenging behaviors in ASD may help to elucidate the meaning, origin, and impact of such behaviors and clarify whether behaviors are part of a comorbid psychiatric presentation requiring targeted management [20] (see Chapter 6).

The use of diagnostic interviews and symptom rating scales may help to highlight the presence of psychiatric symptoms in ASD, and direct further questioning on history to distinguish whether symptoms have consistently been part of the clinical presentation (ie, present since early childhood) or if symptoms have recently emerged, or worsened and are associated with additional impairment and may now be indicative of a comorbid psychiatric disorder. Once psychiatric symptoms have been identified as present in individuals with ASD, careful attention must be paid to whether symptoms contribute significantly to impairment over and above impairment caused by core symptoms of ASD. For identification and characterization of episodic psychiatric disorders (such as anxiety and mood disorders), it is important to first establish symptoms/behaviors that are chronically present in an individual with ASD and part of the baseline clinical presentation (ie, restricted interests, repetitive behavior, baseline affect). These baseline symptoms/behaviors can then be distinguished from the onset of new ones, which may represent an episodic change in presentation representative of a comorbid psychiatric disorder. Once new onset symptoms/behaviors are identified, their duration, relationship with recent stressors (ie, a new teacher, change in environment), and effect on functioning can be assessed.

The Schedule for the Assessment of Psychiatric Problems Associated with Autism (and Other Developmental Disorders [SAPPA]) is one instrument developed to assist clinicians in distinguishing between episodes of behavioral change in ASD that may represent psychiatric comorbidity versus behaviors that are part of the background clinical presentation [21,22]. As some evidence indicates that children with ASD may be particularly sensitive to environmental context, resulting in varying presentations of psychopathology in different settings (ie, school vs. home), particularly for mood and anxiety symptoms, clinicians must be cautious around drawing conclusions regarding diagnosis based on a single informant [23]. Obtaining collateral information from teachers, therapists, or peers (in adults) is invaluable to the process of clarifying whether comorbid psychiatric symptoms interfere significantly with functioning across different contexts and meet criteria for diagnosis of a comorbid disorder.

Clinical pearls for distinguishing between autism spectrum disorder symptoms and common psychiatric symptoms

Social anxiety versus impaired social interaction/communication in autism spectrum disorder

Social anxiety disorder is defined in the DSM-5 as a marked fear or anxiety around social situations that involve potential exposure to scrutiny by peers [4]. In individuals with ASD, it is necessary to look for or inquire about specific changes in behavior/levels of physiological arousal when a person is engaging in a social interaction, being observed, or performing in front of others. Signs of social anxiety in individuals with ASD may include a change in eye contact, facial expressions, and gestures from the individual's *typical* style of social interaction in familiar situations. In comorbid social anxiety disorder, signs of physiological arousal may be present in social situations (ie, shaking, sweating, increased heart rate, shortness of breath) but not at baseline. Further, social situations may be avoided by the affected individual despite a desire to meet new people.

Obsessive compulsive disorder versus repetitive ritualistic behaviors

In the DSM-5, obsessions are defined as persistent unwanted and intrusive thoughts, urges, or image that cause distress or anxiety and attempts are made to ignore/suppress, or neutralize them with some other thought or action [4]. Compulsions are defined as repetitive behaviors or mental acts that an individual feels driven to perform:

- in response to an obsession or according to rules that must be applied rigidly; and
- to prevent or reduce anxiety [4].

In evaluating impairment caused by repetitive behaviors in the context of OCD, compulsions must take up a significant portion of time (>1 hour/day) or cause significant distress/impairment in social, occupational, or other areas of functioning in order to meet criteria for an OCD diagnosis [4]. Although higher functioning adolescents and adults with ASD may be able to articulate the aims of repetitive behaviors, it may not be possible in lower functioning individuals or young children with ASD. Repetitive thoughts and behaviors are both a core feature of OCD and ASD and, as a result, are difficult to distinguish clinically [17]. However, some evidence suggests that the quality and content of repetitive thoughts and behaviors in ASD differ significantly from symptoms typically found in OCD and can be used to help distinguish between the two disorders. These behaviors are summarized in Table 3.1 [24].

Clarifying the onset, quality, and course of repetitive behaviors in individuals with ASD may help to indicate whether repetitive behaviors

Obsessive compulsive disorder	Autism spectrum disorder
Aggression	Repetitive ordering
Contamination	Hoarding
Sexual content	Telling or asking
Symmetry	Touching
Cleaning	Tapping
Checking	Rubbing
Counting	Self-damaging/self-mutilation

Table 3.1 Comparison of obsessive and repetitive behaviors commonly found in obsessive compulsive disorder and autism spectrum disorder.

have always been a part of the presentation, if the quality of behaviors have changed or new onset behaviors has emerged, or that they may be part of a comorbid OCD presentation.

Treating comorbid anxiety disorders

Clinical trials examining the efficacy of psychopharmacological interventions for anxiety symptoms in ASD have yet to be published. Therefore, the use of medications, such as selective serotonin reuptake inhibitors (SSRIs), usually indicated in typically developing populations for anxiety symptoms [25], is currently off-label in ASD. Several randomized controlled trials (RCTs) have examined the use of modified cognitive behavioral therapy (CBT) for treatment of anxiety in children and adolescents with high functioning ASD [26–30]. CBT programs applied to ASD follow general principles [1,27,29,30]:

- affect recognition training;
- the use of relaxation strategies;
- cognitive restructuring;
- graded exposure;
- parent-training component to teach parents to provide support; and
- positive reinforcement and encouragement of independence in children

Increased use of visual supports and predictability of routine in treatment sessions, use of reward, and incorporation of children's circumscribed interests into concept training are often included in CBT programs modified for use in ASD to improve participant motivation [1,27,29,30]. Published studies (n=40–70; age range=7–14 years) that have included a parent component in CBT treatment have demonstrated an approximately 50–75% response rate in participants with comorbid social, separation, generalized anxiety disorder, and OCD over 12–16 weeks of treatment, with maintenance of treatment gains demonstrated at 3- and 6-month follow-up [27,29,30].

Assessing attention deficit hyperactivity disorder symptoms in autism spectrum disorder

As rates of comorbid ADHD are high among individuals with ASD, and individuals with ASD have been shown to respond to stimulant medications [31], a careful assessment for symptoms of inattention, hyperactivity, and impulsivity is essential for treatment planning. In ASD, individuals may be able to attend for prolonged periods of time when engaged in preferred activities, but may struggle with inattention overall. Therefore, it is important to consider an individual's ability to attend to both preferred and non-preferred tasks. As in the non-ASD population, the use of objective rating scales [32] can be used to assess for the presence and severity of ADHD symptoms across two settings in individuals with ASD. If symptoms meet criteria for ADHD, a comorbid diagnosis should be made.

Treating comorbid attention deficit hyperactivity disorder

To date, a small number of RCTs have examined the efficacy of psychotropic medications for treatment of inattention, hyperactivity, and impulsivity in ASD [31]. Two large studies have found the atypical antipsychotic, risperidone, to be superior to placebo for treatment of hyperactivity in children and adolescents with ASD aged 5–17 years [33,34].

Two additional large trials demonstrated the superiority of a second atypical antipsychotic, aripiprazole, for the treatment of hyperactivity in children and adolescents 6–18 years of age, with ASD [35,36]. Although, there is some evidence for the efficacy of atypical antipsychotics for treatment of ADHD symptoms in ASD, these medications are associated with significant adverse effects (eg, weight gain, metabolic effects) and should only be initiated following careful consideration with families around the costs and benefits of treatment and in the context of close metabolic monitoring [20].

Two RCTs in children aged 5–14 years examined the efficacy of the stimulant methylphenidate as treatment for ADHD symptoms in ASD and reported a 50% response rate for symptoms of hyperactivity, inattention, and impulsivity [37]; however, significant adverse effects were cause for discontinuation in 18% of those treated [38,39]. Therefore, methylphenidate treatment may be efficacious for treatment of ADHD symptoms in ASD, but individuals with ASD may be less responsive than those with a primary ADHD diagnosis and more sensitive to side effects [31].

One relatively large RCT [40] and one smaller placebo crossover trial [41] (n=16–97; age range=6–17 years; IQ>60) examined the efficacy of atomoxetine, a norepinephrine reuptake inhibitor, for ADHD symptoms in ASD. Both demonstrated moderate improvement in symptoms of inattention, hyperactivity, and impulsivity in treated children when compared to placebo [40,41]. Atomoxetine was generally well tolerated with no significant adverse effects reported [40,41].

Assessing for depressive symptoms in autism spectrum disorder

Rates of major depressive disorder may increase with age and some evidence suggests that prevalence may be higher in higher functioning individuals with ASD [19]. In the DSM, major depressive disorder is defined by a marked change from previous functioning that is accompanied by either the presence of depressed mood or loss of interest or pleasure (anhedonia) in all or almost all activities, with symptoms that are present most of the day, nearly every day, for two weeks or more [4].

In order to meet criteria for major depressive disorder, depressed mood or anhedonia must be accompanied by four additional symptoms over the same two-week period, such as:

- change in eating/weight;
- lower energy levels;
- altered sleep patterns;
- trouble with concentration;
- psychomotor changes;

- feelings of worthlessness and guilt; and/or
- recurrent thoughts of death or suicidal ideation.

Obtaining evidence of a change in mood or levels of interest/pleasure in activities from baseline is key to assessing for the presence of major depression in ASD. According to a recent review of studies describing phenomenology of depression in ASD, depressed mood has frequently been found in individuals with ASD and comorbid depression, though it is most often reported by a third party as opposed to the affected individual [42]. Anhedonia may manifest as a decrease in repetitive behavior or the usual intensity of circumscribed interests. Decreased self-care may be observed and new onset or exacerbation of maladaptive (including aggressive or oppositional) behaviors may emerge [1]. Therefore, obtaining history from a third party and focusing on change in observable behaviors may help to appropriately identify depression in ASD.

Treating comorbid depression

There are currently no published studies to guide treatment of depression in children and adolescents with ASD. A recent preliminary study of a modified mindfulness-based therapy protocol for high functioning adults with ASD has shown some promise for treatment of depressive symptoms in this population; however, more research examining the efficacy of common treatments for depression (ie, SSRIs, CBT for depressive symptoms) in the ASD population is needed [43].

Conclusions

Psychiatric comorbidity is common in ASD and must be part of the general assessment of affected individuals and considered when developing a treatment plan. Recent changes in the DSM-5 now facilitate the diagnosis of comorbid psychiatric conditions in ASD. However, there are very few validated tools to help support clinicians in assessing for comorbid disorders in this population. Therefore, clinicians must use psychiatric tools with caution when assessing for psychiatric comorbidity in ASD, and use their clinical judgment in combination with direct observation of the affected individual, careful history taking with parents/caregivers, family, and collateral information obtained from other relevant informants (ie, teachers, therapists) to determine whether a comorbid psychiatric diagnosis should be made. Currently, treatment of psychiatric conditions in ASD is often based on findings regarding treatment efficacy in non-ASD populations. Improved identification of psychiatric comorbidity in ASD may help to drive assessment and treatment research in this important clinical area.

References

1 Kim JA, Szatmari P, Bryson SE, Wilson FJ. The prevalence of anxiety and mood problems among children with autism and asperger syndrome. *Autism.* 2000;4:117-132.

2 Johnson CP, Myers SM. Identification and evaluation of children with autism spectrum disorders. *Pediatrics.* 2007;120:1183-1215.

3 American Psychiatric Association. *Diagnostic and Statistical Manual of Mental Disorders.* 4th edn, Text Revision. Washington, DC: American Psychiatric Association; 2000.

4 American Psychiatric Association. *Diagnostic and Statistical Manual of Mental Disorders.* 5th edn. Washington, DC: American Psychiatric Association; 2013.

5 Abdallah MW, Greaves-Lord K, Grove J, Norgaard-Pedersen B, Hougaard DM, Mortensen EL. Psychiatric comorbidities in autism spectrum disorders: findings from a Danish Historic Birth Cohort. *Eur Child Adolesc Psychiatry.* 2011; 20:599-601.

6 Leyfer OT, Folstein SE, Bacalman S, et al. Comorbid psychiatric disorders in children with autism: interview development and rates of disorders. *J Autism Dev Disord.* 2006;36:849-861.

7 Simonoff E, Pickles A, Charman T, Chandler S, Loucas T, Baird G. Psychiatric disorders in children with autism spectrum disorders: prevalence, comorbidity, and associated factors in a population-derived sample. *J Am Acad Child Adolesc Psychiatry.* 2008;47:921-929.

8 van Steensel FJ, Bogels SM, Perrin S. Anxiety disorders in children and adolescents with autistic spectrum disorders: a meta-analysis. *Clin Child Fam Psychol Rev.* 2011;14:302-317.

9 Mattila ML, Kielinen M, Linna SL, et al. Autism spectrum disorders according to DSM-IV-TR and comparison with DSM-5 draft criteria: an epidemiological study. *J Am Acad Child Adolesc Psychiatry.* 2011;50:583-592 e511.

10 Skokauskas N, Gallagher L. Mental health aspects of autistic spectrum disorders in children. *J Intellect Disabil Res.* 2012;56:248-257.

11 Mattila ML, Hurtig T, Haapsamo H, et al. Comorbid psychiatric disorders associated with Asperger syndrome/high-functioning autism: a community- and clinic-based study. *J Autism Dev Disord.* 2010;40:1080-1093.

12 Maskey M, Warnell F, Parr JR, Le Couteur A, McConachie H. Emotional and behavioural problems in children with autism spectrum disorder. *J Autism Dev Disord.* 2013;43:851-859.

13 Hofvander B, Delorme R, Chaste P, et al. Psychiatric and psychosocial problems in adults with normal-intelligence autism spectrum disorders. *BMC Psychiatry.* 2009;9:35.

14 Lugnegard T, Hallerback MU, Gillberg C. Personality disorders and autism spectrum disorders: what are the connections? *Compr Psychiatry.* 2012;53:333-340.

15 Melville CA, Cooper SA, Morrison J, et al. The prevalence and incidence of mental ill-health in adults with autism and intellectual disabilities. *J Autism Dev Disord.* 2008;38:1676-1688.

16 Weisbrot DM, Gadow KD, DeVincent CJ, Pomeroy J. The presentation of anxiety in children with pervasive developmental disorders. *J Child Adolesc Psychopharmacol.* 2005;15:477-496.

17 Mazzone L, Ruta L, Reale L. Psychiatric comorbidities in asperger syndrome and high functioning autism: diagnostic challenges. *Ann Gen Psychiatry.* 2012;11:16.

18 Practice parameter for the assessment and treatment of children and adolescents with autism spectrum disorder. *J Am Acad Child Adolesc Psychiatry.* 2014;53:237-257.

19 Sterling L, Dawson G, Estes A, Greenson J. Characteristics associated with presence of depressive symptoms in adults with autism spectrum disorder. *J Autism Dev Disord.* 2008;38:1011-1018.

20 Ameis SH, Corbett-Dick P, Cole L, Correll CU. Decision making and antipsychotic medication treatment for youth with autism spectrum disorders: applying guidelines in the real world. *J Clin Psychiatry.* 2013;74:1022-1024.

21 Bolton PFRM. *Schedule for Assessment of Psychiatric Problems Associated with Ausitm (And other Developmental Disorders (SAPPA): Informant Version.*: Cambridge: University of Cambridge; London: Institute of Psychiatry; 1994.

22 Bradley E, Bolton P. Episodic psychiatric disorders in teenagers with learning disabilities with and without autism. *Br J Psychiatry.* 2006;189:361-366.

23 Kanne SM, Abbacchi AM, Constantino JN. Multi-informant ratings of psychiatric symptom severity in children with autism spectrum disorders: the importance of environmental context. *J Autism Dev Disord.* 2009;39:856-864.

24 McDougle CJ, Kresch LE, Goodman WK, et al. A case-controlled study of repetitive thoughts and behavior in adults with autistic disorder and obsessive-compulsive disorder. *Am J Psychiatry.*1995;152:772-777.

25 Connolly SD, Bernstein GA. Practice parameter for the assessment and treatment of children and adolescents with anxiety disorders. *J Am Acad Child Adolesc Psychiatry.* 2007;46:267-283.

26 Chalfant AM, Rapee R, Carroll L. Treating anxiety disorders in children with high functioning autism spectrum disorders: a controlled trial. *J Autism Dev Disord.* 2007;37:1842-1857.

27 Reaven J, Blakeley-Smith A, Leuthe E, Moody E, Hepburn S. Facing your fears in adolescence: cognitive-behavioral therapy for high-functioning autism spectrum disorders and anxiety. *Autism Res Treat.* 2012;2012:423905.

28 Sofronoff K, Attwood T, Hinton S, Levin I. A randomized controlled trial of a cognitive behavioural intervention for anger management in children diagnosed with Asperger syndrome. *J Autism Dev Disord.* 2007;37:1203-1214.

29 Storch EA, Arnold EB, Lewin AB, et al. The effect of cognitive-behavioral therapy versus treatment as usual for anxiety in children with autism spectrum disorders: a randomized, controlled trial. *J Am Acad Child Adolesc Psychiatry.* 2013;52:132-142 e132.

30 Wood JJ, Drahota A, Sze K, Har K, Chiu A, Langer DA. Cognitive behavioral therapy for anxiety in children with autism spectrum disorders: a randomized, controlled trial. *J Child Psychol Psychiatry.* 2009;50:224-234.

31 Reichow B, Volkmar FR, Bloch MH. Systematic review and meta-analysis of pharmacological treatment of the symptoms of attention-deficit/hyperactivity disorder in children with pervasive developmental disorders. *J Autism Dev Disord.* 2013;43:2435-2441.

32 Lakes KD, Swanson JM, Riggs M. The reliability and validity of the English and Spanish Strengths and Weaknesses of ADHD and Normal behavior rating scales in a preschool sample: continuum measures of hyperactivity and inattention. *J Atten Disord.* 2012;16:510-516.

33 McCracken JT, McGough J, Shah B, et al. Risperidone in children with autism and serious behavioral problems. *N Engl J Med.* 2002;347:314-321.

34 Shea S, Turgay A, Carroll A, et al. Risperidone in the treatment of disruptive behavioral symptoms in children with autistic and other pervasive developmental disorders. *Pediatrics.* 2004;114:e634-641.

35 Marcus RN, Owen R, Kamen L, et al. A placebo-controlled, fixed-dose study of aripiprazole in children and adolescents with irritability associated with autistic disorder. *J Am Acad Child Adolesc Psychiatry.* 2009;48:1110-1119.

36 Owen R, Sikich L, Marcus RN, et al. Aripiprazole in the treatment of irritability in children and adolescents with autistic disorder. *Pediatrics.* 2009;124:1533-1540.

37 Randomized, controlled, crossover trial of methylphenidate in pervasive developmental disorders with hyperactivity. *Arch Gen Psychiatry.* 2005;62:1266-1274.

38 Abikoff H, McGough J, Vitiello B, et al. Sequential pharmacotherapy for children with comorbid attention-deficit/hyperactivity and anxiety disorders. *J Am Acad Child Adolesc Psychiatry.* 2005;44:418-427.

39 Handen BL, Johnson CR, Lubetsky M. Efficacy of methylphenidate among children with autism and symptoms of attention-deficit hyperactivity disorder. *J Autism Dev Disord.* 2000;30:245-255.

40 Harfterkamp M, van de Loo-Neus G, Minderaa RB, et al. A randomized double-blind study of atomoxetine versus placebo for attention-deficit/hyperactivity disorder symptoms in children with autism spectrum disorder. *J Am Acad Child Adolesc Psychiatry.* 2012;51:733-741.

41 Arnold LE, Aman MG, Cook AM, et al. Atomoxetine for hyperactivity in autism spectrum disorders: placebo-controlled crossover pilot trial. *J Am Acad Child Adolesc Psychiatry.* 2006;45:1196-1205.

42 Stewart ME, Barnard L, Pearson J, Hasan R, O'Brien G. Presentation of depression in autism and Asperger syndrome: a review. *Autism.* 2006;10:103-116.

43 Spek AA, van Ham NC, Nyklicek I. Mindfulness-based therapy in adults with an autism spectrum disorder: a randomized controlled trial. *Res Dev Disabil.* 2013;34:246-253.

Chapter 4

Medical comorbidities in autism spectrum disorder

Jennifer R Walton and Daniel L Coury

Key Learning Objectives

By the end of this chapter, readers will be able to:

- describe commonly co-occurring medical conditions in autism spectrum disorder (ASD);
- recognize that gastrointestinal (GI) conditions occur commonly in ASD and can cause significant changes in behavior;
- identify genetic conditions commonly associated with ASD;
- describe evidence-based treatments for sleep problems in individuals with ASD; and
- effectively screen for co-occurring medical conditions through increased awareness and changes in clinical practice.

Introduction

ASD is a behaviorally defined neurodevelopmental disorder. As the term spectrum implies, it refers to a heterogeneous group of phenotypes with a range of neurobiologic features. Some cases occur in other medical conditions such as Fragile X syndrome; in such instances, medical comorbidities are usually seen as part of the underlying medical disorder. In ASD that is not associated with a known medical syndrome, conditions such as epilepsy, GI dysfunction, and sleep disorders occur more frequently than in the general population [1]. These medical conditions occurring in

E. Anagnostou and J. Brian (eds.), *Clinician's Manual on Autism Spectrum Disorder*, DOI 10.1007/978-3-319-03056-2_4

patients with a primary diagnosis of ASD may simply represent the fact that people with ASD can also have other medical disorders. However, others may represent part of a yet to be defined autism subtype, such as is suggested by the association of certain mesenchymal-epithelial transition factor (MET) gene polymorphisms with GI disorders in some individuals with ASD [2].

Whatever the precise relationship, identification and treatment of medical conditions in individuals with ASD is an important part of an overall management program. This chapter will discuss the more commonly co-occurring medical conditions and suggestions for treatment.

Epilepsy

Epilepsy has been reported to occur in approximately 7–35% of patients with ASD [3,4]. Seizures are noted most commonly in the first 2–5 years of life and are sometimes diagnosed concurrently with ASD. The lifetime risk increases during adolescence, especially in patients with ASD and intellectual disability (ID). A recent meta-analysis described a pooled prevalence of epilepsy in 21.5% of individuals with ASD and ID, in contrast to 8% in those with ASD without ID [5]. These findings demonstrate that the prevalence of epilepsy is considerably higher in individuals with ASD and ID than in those with ASD alone, with overall rates more than ten times that of the non-ASD population.

Epilepsy and ASD may co-occur because of common pathophysiologic mechanisms related to abnormal synaptic plasticity and altered excitation/inhibition ratios in the developing brain [4]. In fact, several single gene disorders associated with both ASD and epilepsy, such as Fragile X syndrome or tuberous sclerosis, are known to be associated with pathways such as glutamate and γ-aminobutyric acid (GABA). On the other hand, early seizures in the developing brain may lead to alterations in synaptic plasticity and contribute to the development of ASD. For example, the synapsin genes regulate neurotransmitter release and short-term synaptic plasticity and have been associated with both epilepsy and ASD [6]. This has led to experimental models of ASD in genetically-modified knockout mice.

Individuals with ASD may present with variety of seizure types including grand mal and petit mal. Partial complex seizures reportedly occur most often, but can be difficult to assess. This is because the movements seen in partial complex seizures can be confused with the repetitive and unusual motor behaviors often seen as part of the behavioral presentation of ASD. Clinicians should be alert to changes in motor behaviors and mental status in these patients as these may be subtle signs of seizures.

Impact of epilepsy in autism spectrum disorder

Some types of epilepsy in ASD are associated with regression in social, language, and motor skills. While this is seen most often in younger patients (eg, epileptic encephalopathies of infancy and childhood), it can also be seen in adolescents. The fairly abrupt onset of regression in these individuals generally leads to lengthy evaluation, which typically includes electroencephalography (EEG) and imaging studies, genomic testing, and a metabolic genetics evaluation. Controversy remains around the implications of active epileptiform EEGs in the absence of clinical seizures. Current guidelines do not recommend routine use of screening EEGs in children with ASD [7]. However, a high degree of clinical suspicion for epilepsy should be maintained for children with regression in language or social communication, especially in those older than 3 years of age with language regression.

Treatment of epilepsy in autism spectrum disorder

Although the potential shared biology between epilepsy and ASD should have implications for choice of therapeutic agents, at this point, anticonvulsants have not been studied with respected to seizure cessation efficacy in ASD. Thus, treatment in this population remains the same as for individuals without autism (eg, anticonvulsants).

Gastrointestinal conditions

GI symptoms are common in the general population, although there has been controversy over their precise prevalence in the ASD population. Studies have shown that there are higher reports of GI symptoms in the ASD population, as well as in other populations of individuals with neurodevelopmental disorders, than in the general population [8]. In a prospective study, Valicenti-McDermott et al identified GI symptoms (eg, frequent vomiting, prior diagnosis of gastroesophageal reflux, abdominal pain, abnormal stool pattern, characteristics of the bowel movement and constipation) in 70% of their sample with ASD, versus 42% in a developmentally disabled group, and 28% in typically developing children [8]. When identified, there has been controversy over the underlying cause and appropriate treatment for these problems. Studies suggesting unique autism-related pathology have been largely retracted or dismissed [9]. On the other hand, children and adolescents with ASD report common GI conditions such as chronic constipation or diarrhea, gastroesophageal reflux (GERD), and inflammatory bowel disease. These generally present with the same symptoms as are seen in typically developing individuals, although they may be harder to detect in children with limited communication abilities. However, families have reported difficulty convincing their health care provider to conduct appropriate evaluations [10]. A thorough review of the literature related to GI conditions in ASD has provided recommendations for treatment [11]. The strongest recommendation is for clinicians to listen to families' concerns and evaluate and treat GI symptoms in individuals with ASD the same way as in typically developing children.

An important point to highlight is that, because of the core deficits in social communication and possibly due to some sensory abnormalities, individuals with ASD may have GI symptoms that do not manifest in typical ways, but instead may appear as unusual behaviors. There have been reports of individuals with writhing and aggressive behaviors originally interpreted as being associated with underlying autism, but that were later identified as being more similar to Sandifer syndrome [12]. This syndrome of GI disease and dystonic body movements responds well to treatment of the underlying GI condition, rather than medical treatment of the presenting behaviors. Clinicians should be thorough in their history-taking and consider further investigation for possible medical explanations for behavior changes.

More recent studies are identifying abnormalities in gut microbiota associated with autism [13]. The full significance of these findings, and any potential treatment for them, has yet to be determined.

Sleep issues

The importance of sleep for overall health is well known. However, studies have shown that the prevalence of sleep difficulties in the ASD population range from 44–86%, compared to 20–30% in the general population [14]. Kotagal and Broomall provide a detailed review of developmental aspects of sleep dysregulation in ASD [15]. For example, a reduction in GABA receptors in anterior and posterior cingulate gyri, which are important in social-emotional processing, has been reported in ASD, leading to the suggestion that there may be a relationship between reduced GABA receptors in the cingulate cortex and the disruption of initiating and maintaining sleep in individuals with ASD. Alteration in the release of melatonin has also been suggested as a possible mechanism for disrupted sleep in ASD. Sleep difficulties are not influenced by the type of ASD or level of cognitive impairment, but there may be a correlation between sleep difficulties and aggressive behavior, developmental regression, and internalizing problems such as anxiety [15].

A variety of sleep disorders occur in the ASD population, with insomnia being most commonly reported [14]. Per the American Academy of Sleep Medicine's diagnostic and coding manual, components of insomnia include:

- difficulty initiating or maintaining sleep;
- waking up too early and not being able to return to sleep; and
- insufficient or poor quality sleep [16].

In the ASD patient population, the cause of insomnia is multifactorial; usually it is behavior-based, but there are other possible causes that need to be ruled out, including neurologic, respiratory, and psychiatric conditions [17]. These include obstructive sleep apnea, obesity, epilepsy, anxiety, and attention-deficit hyperactivity disorder (ADHD).

The process of identifying, evaluating, and managing insomnia and other sleep disorders in the ASD population is important and should be thorough [15,17]. First, it is important that these individuals are always screened, either through a questionnaire/checklist or a detailed sleep history. Questions to pursue include the length of time it takes for a child to fall asleep, how long the child sleeps, if there are night-time awakenings, description of daytime naps, whether the child is taking medications that may affect sleep or overall alertness, and if there are daytime behaviors of concern (inattentiveness, mood swings) [15,17].

Second, the health care provider should identify any other contributors that may relate to sleep dysfunction (including neurologic, GI, or psychiatric conditions) and determine if they are causing the disruption [17]. Lastly, the provider should work with the family in planning an intervention to manage the sleep difficulties.

Interventions for sleep disorders in autism spectrum disorder

Educational and behavioral interventions to improve sleep hygiene are considered first-line treatment. Behavioral interventions used in typically developing children are frequently effective, but require more attention to parent training and support [17,18]. For those individuals with ASD who have insomnia or delayed sleep-phase syndrome, melatonin has been shown to be effective [19]. Supplemental melatonin has been shown to improve sleep latency, as measured by actigraphy, in most children at 1 or 3 mg dosages; effectiveness can be seen in week 1 of treatment and is maintained for several months [19]. It is well tolerated, safe, and showed additional benefits for behavior and parenting stress [19]. Melatonic has also become widely used as an initial medical treatment in individuals without ASD.

Restless legs syndrome (RLS) is a disorder that can affect individuals with ASD and is characterized by poor sleep, frequent lower extremity movements, and commonly, a family history of similar symptoms. In cases of pediatric RLS, oral iron has been found to be effective, with approximately 80% of the subjects given supplemental iron showing improvement or resolution of their symptoms within 4 months of beginning treatment [20].

In patients presenting with anxiety, clonidine, guanfacine, and selective serotonin reuptake inhibitors (SSRIs) have been trialled [15]. However, currently there is limited evidence for the use of medications to treat insomnia in children with ASD [17].

Associated genetic syndromes

Currently, the molecular basis for ASD can be identified in 10–20% of cases [21]. Findings to date indicate that genetic contributions to autism are highly heterogeneous. More than 200 loci have been found to confer risk of ASD in different individuals, although each variation accounts for less than 1% of individuals with ASD. In addition, the phenotypic expression or penetrance of these genetic components is also highly variable. Studies have demonstrated a range from fully penetrant point mutations to polygenic forms with multiple gene-gene and gene-environment interactions [22,23].

In 10% of individuals with ASD, an associated medical condition or syndrome can be identified [24]. This includes such syndromes as:

- Fragile X;
- neurocutaneous disorders (such as tuberous sclerosis);
- phenylketonuria;
- fetal alcohol syndrome;
- Angelman syndrome;
- Rett syndrome;
- Smith-Lemli-Opitz syndrome;
- Down's syndrome; and
- Coloboma, Heart defect, Atresia choanae, Retarded growth and development, Genital abnormality, and Ear abnormality (CHARGE) syndrome.

Other recently identified syndromic autisms are associated with chromosomal variations at 1q21, 15q13, and 16p11.2 [25]. Primary care providers who have patients with these syndromes should evaluate them for the presence of ASD characteristics. Conversely, patients with diagnosed ASD should undergo genetic testing to rule out other possible syndromes.

Currently, the American College of Medical Genetics recommends a chromosomal microarray as a first-line assessment in individuals diagnosed with ASD, along with testing for Fragile X [26]. Specific testing for other associated syndromes may be ordered based on level of suspicion.

In addition to associated single gene disorders, genetic testing may be fruitful in the future to reveal associations between ASD and other medical comorbidities. For example, the *MET rs1858830 C* allele, which is important to both brain development and gastrointestinal repair has been found to be overrepresented in families with co-occurring ASD and GI conditions [27].

Conclusions

Individuals with ASD may present with a variety of medical conditions, some simply co-occurring, and some likely associated with their underlying biology. A careful history is still the most import clinical tool, with special attention paid to conditions which are known to be present in high frequency, such as epilepsy, GI dysfunction, and sleep problems. Further research into potential common biology between ASD symptoms and medical comorbidities, as is the case for the MET polymorphism, will hopefully clarify the question of which conditions are simply co-occurring and which highlight specific subgroupings within ASD. Continued education for primary care providers for patients with ASD and other comorbidities is critical, as these patients will need to receive comprehensive, coordinated, and community-based care.

References

1 Coury DL. Medical treatment of autism spectrum disorders. *Curr Opin Neurol.* 2010;23:131-136.

2 Campbell DB1, Buie TM, Winter H, Bauman M, Sutcliffe JS, Perrin JM, Levitt P. Distinct genetic risk based on association of MET in families with co-occurring autism and gastrointestinal conditions. *Pediatrics.* 2009;123:1018-1024.

3 Minshew, NJ, Sweeney JA, Bauman ML. Neurologic aspects of autism. In, Cohen DJ, Volkmar FR, eds. *Handbook of Autism and Pervasive Developmental Disorders.* 2nd edn. New York, New York: Wiley; 1997.

4 Tuchman R, Hirtz D, Mamounas LA. NINDS epilepsy and autism spectrum disorders workshop report. *Neurology* 2013;81;1630-1636.

5 Amiet C, Gourfinkel-An I, Bouzamondo A, et al. Epilepsy in autism is associated with intellectual disability and gender: evidence from a meta-analysis. *Biol Psychiatry.* 2008;64:577-582.

6 Giovedí S, Corradi A, Fassio A, Benfenati F. Involvement of synaptic genes in the pathogenesis of autism spectrum disorders: the case of synapsins. *Front Pediatr.* 2014;2:94.

7 Kagan-Kushnir T, Roberts SW, Snead 3rd OC. Screening electroencephalograms in autism spectrum disorders: evidence based guideline. *J Child Neurol.* 2005;20:197-206.

8 Valicenti-McDermott M, McVicar K, Rapin I, Wershil BK, Cohen H, Shinnar S. Frequency of gastrointestinal symptoms in children with autistic spectrum disorders and association with family history of autoimmune disease. *J Dev Behav Pediatrics.* 2006; 27;S128-S136.

9 Wakefield AJ, Murch SH, Anthony A, et al. Ileal-lymphoid-nodular hyperplasia, non-specific colitis, and pervasive developmental disorder in children. *Lancet.* 1998;35:637-641. Retraction in: *Lancet.* 2010;375:445. Partial retraction in: Murch SH, Anthony A, Casson DH, Malik M, et al. *Lancet.* 2004;363:750.

10 Carbone PS, Behl DD, Azor V, Murphy NA. The medical home for children with autism spectrum disorders: parent and pediatrician perspectives. *J Autism Dev Disord.* 2010;40:317-324.

11 Buie T, Fuchs GJ 3rd, Furuta GT, et al. Recommendations for evaluation and treatment of common gastrointestinal problems in children with ASDs. *Pediatrics.* 2010;125(suppl 1):S19-S29.

12 Lehwald N, Krausch M, Franke C, Assmann B, Adam R, Knoefel WT. Sandifer syndrome--a multidisciplinary diagnostic and therapeutic challenge. *Eur J Pediatr Surg.* 2007;17:203-206.

13 Williams BL, Hornig M, Buie T, et al. Impaired carbohydrate digestion and transport and mucosal dysbiosis in the intestines of children with autism and gastrointestinal disturbances. *PLoS One.* 2011;6:e24585.

14 Porter AE, Glaze DG. Sleep Problems. In, Amaral D, Dawson G, Geschwind D, eds, *Autism Spectrum Disorders.* Oxford, UK: Oxford University Press; 2011.

15 Kotagal S, Broomall E. Sleep in children with autism spectrum disorder. *Pediatr Neurol.* 2012;47:242-225.

16 American Academy of Sleep Medicine. *International Classification of Sleep Disorders, Diagnostic and Coding Manual.* 2nd edn. Westchester, IL: American Academy of Sleep Medicine; 2005.

17 Malow BA, Byars K, Johnson K, et al. A practice pathway for the identification, evaluation, and management of insomnia in children and adolescents with autism spectrum disorders. *Pediatrics.* 2012;130:S106-S124.

18 Malow BA, Adkins KW, Reynolds A, etal T. Parent-based sleep education for children with autism spectrum disorders. *J Autism Dev Disord.* 2014;44:216-228.

19 Malow B, Adkins KW, McGrew SG, et al. Melatonin for sleep in children with autism: a controlled trial examining dose, tolerability, and outcomes. *J Autism Dev Disord.* 2012;42:1729-1737.

20 Amos LB, Grekowicz ML, Kuhn EM, et al. Treatment of pediatric restless legs syndrome. *Clin Pediatr (Phila).* 2014;53:331-336.

21 Geschwind D. Commentary: autism genetics and genomics: a brief overview and synthesis. In, Amaral D, Dawson G, Geschwind D, eds. *Autism Spectrum Disorders.* Oxford, UK : Oxford University Press; 2011.

22 Sebat J, Lakshmi B, Malhotra D, et al. Strong association of de novo copy number mutations with autism. *Science.* 2007;316 :445-449.

23 Klei L, Sanders SJ, Murtha MT, et al. Common genetic variants, acting additively, are a major source of risk for autism. *Mol Autism.* 2012;3:9.

24 Johnson CP, Myers SM. Identification and evaluation of children with autism spectrum disorders. *Pediatrics.* 2007;120:1183-1215.

25 Persico AM, Napolioni V. Autism genetics. *Behav Brain Res.* 2013 251:95-112.

26 Miller DT, Adam MP, Aradhya S, Biesecker LG, et al. Consensus statement: chromosomal microarray is a first-tier clinical diagnostic test for individuals with developmental disabilities or congenital anomalies. *Am J Hum Genet.* 2010;86:749-764.

27 Campbell DB, Buie TM, Winter H, et al. Distinct genetic risk based on association of MET in families with co-occurring autism and gastrointestinal conditions. *Pediatrics.* 2009;123:1018-1024.

Chapter 5

Pharmacotherapy in autism spectrum disorder

Sharon Smile, Evdokia Anagnostou

Key Learning Objectives

By the end of this chapter, readers will be able to:

- describe the evidence for commonly prescribed medications in autism spectrum disorder (ASD);
- identify common adverse events; and
- be familiar with monitoring recommendations.

Introduction

ASD is a complex and heterogeneous disorder which is defined by the constellation of impairment in reciprocal social interactions, functional communication skills, and the presence of repetitive and restricted patterns of behavior and interests. Its etiology is still elusive, although a strong genetic component has been documented and gene-environment interactions have been hypothesized. Currently, only behavioral or psychosocial treatments have evidence of benefit for core symptom domains. Pharmacotherapy is one modality of intervention geared at removing barriers to learning by targeting associated symptoms of ASD such as irritability, aggression, and attention deficit hyperactive disorder (ADHD) symptoms, among others. It is important to ensure that fundamental interventions, such as behavioral programs that focus on skill development, are in place prior to or concurrent with pharmacotherapy, thus optimizing the effect of pharmacotherapy.

E. Anagnostou and J. Brian (eds.), *Clinician's Manual on Autism Spectrum Disorder*, DOI 10.1007/978-3-319-03056-2_5

The limited understanding of the pathophysiology of ASD has resulted in the absence of any pharmacological agents that have been derived through the translational route, and as such, no pharmacotherapies have been demonstrated to be effective for core symptom domains. Thus, clinicians use a symptom-based approach to address maladaptive behaviors in ASD. This chapter will review the evidence for such an approach, including recent randomized controlled trials (RCTs) and meta-analyses that support this practice.

Symptom-based approach to the treatment of autism spectrum disorder

With a symptom-based approach, clinicians look for similarities in symptom clusters between ASD and other neuropsychiatric disorders and essentially "borrow" established therapies that are used to treat these other disorders and use them to address the behavioral challenges seen in individuals with ASD. Attention difficulties, impulsivity, hyperactivity, self-injurious behaviors, irritability, repetitive behaviors, anxiety, obsessions, and compulsions are common behaviors exhibited by individuals with ASD.

Hyperactivity, impulsivity, and inattention: attention deficit hyperactivity disorder symptom cluster

The Diagnostic and Statistical Manual of Mental Disorders (DSM-5) diagnostic criteria for ASD now acknowledges that symptoms of hyperactivity, impulsivity, and inattention (in isolation or in combination) are often co-occurring in ASD, and ADHD can now be considered a comorbid diagnosis [1]. Evidence for pharmacotherapy to treat ADHD symptoms associated with ASD is available through clinical trials, as well as meta-analyses, which will be discussed below. There are four main medication categories that are currently used in the management of an ASD/ADHD profile:

- stimulants;
- nonstimulants;
- α2-agonists; and
- antipsychotics.

Regulation of these drugs can vary by country. For example, the US Food and Drug Administration (FDA) and Health Canada have approved the use of stimulants (eg, methylphenidate, amphetamines), one nonstimulant, and $\alpha 2$ agonists (eg, clonidine, guanfacine) for the treatment of ADHD in children generally. Meanwhile, the UK's National Institute for Health and Care Excellence has approved only amphetamines, stimulants, and nonstimulants for the management of ADHD.

Stimulants

Stimulants work centrally to enhance norepinephrine and dopamine transmission through inhibition of dopamine/norepinephrine reuptake in the striatum, among other less understood mechanisms. The two most widely used groups of stimulants include methylphenidate compounds and amphetamines. The best evidence available for stimulants comes from six RCTs of methylphenidate involving preschool and school-aged children with ASD [2–7]. A recent meta-analysis of four of these studies (94 participants collectively) showed that methylphenidate is superior to placebo in treating ADHD symptoms in children with ASD (effect size [ES]=0.67; 95% CI; 0.08–1.27; $P<0.05$), with the strongest effect for hyperactivity in particular (ES =0.66; 95% CI 0.03–1.03; $P<0.001$) [8]. There was also a trend toward methylphenidate decreasing irritability and stereotypic behaviors, but values did not reach statistical significance. The mean dose of methylphenidate used in the studies ranged from 0.29–0.45 mg/kg/dose.

Most recently, Pearson et al [7] demonstrated that the combination of long-acting and immediate-release methylphenidate was associated with a statistically and clinically significant decrease in inattention within the home and school environment, across multiple outcome measures, including:

- Conners' Parent Rating Scale-Revised (CPRS-R) inattention subscale ($P=0.001$) [9];
- Swanson, Noland, and Pelham (SNAP)-IV parent-rated form ($P<0.001$) [10]; and
- Conners' Teacher Rating Scale-Revised (CTRS-R) inattention subscale ($P=0.044$) [11].

This regimen was also associated with reduction in hyperactivity as measured by parents and teachers across multiple outcome measures, including:

- CPRS-R hyperactivity subscale (P=<0.001);
- SNAP-IV parent-rated hyperactivity subscale (P=0.001);
- ADHD Comprehensive Teacher's Rating Scale (ACTeRS) parent hyperactivity subscale (P<0.001);
- CTRS-R hyperactivity subscale (P<0.001) [11];
- SNAP-IV teacher hyperactive subscale (P=0.003) [10]; and
- ACTeRS teacher hyperactivity subscale (P<0.001) [7].

Adverse events of statistical significance frequently reported include decrease in appetite, difficulty falling asleep, irritability, emotional outbursts, and social withdrawal. The response rate of methylphenidate in ASD is reduced compared to children who have ADHD but not ASD (49–60% vs. 70–90%); however, the level of cognitive function does not impact efficacy [12,13].

To date, there have been no RCTs to evaluate the efficacy of amphetamines in children diagnosed with ASD and ADHD. Of note, an early study that explored amphetamine use in schizophrenic children with "autistic features" yielded minimal therapeutic effects [14]; data in children with current or recent definitions of ASD are still pending [15]. The Autism Treatment Network has published a guideline for choosing medications to treat ADHD-like symptoms in children with ASD [16]. Stimulants are recommended as a first-line choice of therapy in children with the ASD/ADHD profile if not contraindicated, followed by atomoxetine and α2-agonists as second-line, and atypical antipsychotics as a third-line choice of therapy [16].

Nonstimulants

Atomoxetine, the only drug in its class with indications for ADHD, is a nonstimulant which selectively inhibits norepinephrine reuptake and has selective dopamine effects in the frontal lobe. There have been two RCTs (one crossover, one parallel design) that support its use in the management of ADHD symptoms in ASD [17,18]. The first, smaller study (n=16) showed improvement of hyperactivity based on both the Aberrant Behavior Checklist (ABC) hyperactivity subscale ($P=0.04$; ES=0.90) and the DSM-IV ADHD impulsivity/hyperactivity symptoms means ($P=0.005$; ES=1.27) [19]. There was also a trend towards decreased inattention ($P=0.053$). In the second, larger study (n=97), atomoxetine resulted in reduced ADHD-Rating Scale scores in the inattention subscore ($P=0.003$) and hyperactivity–impulsivity subscore ($P<0.001$) and reduction in CTRS–RS hyperactivity score ($P=0.024$) [20]. The response rate to atomoxetine in children with ASD was less than that reported in non-ASD children with an ADHD profile (57% vs. 63%) [17,21]. Atomoxetine use is limited by gastrointestinal (GI) symptoms such as nausea, stomach ache, and decreased appetite, as well as early morning awakening and tachycardia.

α2-agonists

Guanfacine functions by stimulating central α2-agonist adrenergic receptors and has been used as a monotherapy to reduce hyperactivity and impulsivity in children. Its efficacy in children with an ASD/ADHD profile has been explored in one small double-blind, placebo-controlled crossover RCT (n=11) with a 45% response rate, whilst titrating up to 3 mg/day dose [22]. Improvements were noted only in hyperactivity on both the Parent and Teacher Aberrant Behavior Checklist (ABC) hyperactivity subscales ($P=0.025$ and $P=0.005$, respectively) [19]. Comparisons in pooled side effect severity between conditions did not meet statistical significance; however, drowsiness, lethargy, irritability, social withdrawal, constipation, and diarrhea were documented in the treatment group.

Clonidine, another α2-agonist, is used as an adjunctive to methylphenidate, as well as monotherapy targeting hyperactivity and impulsivity in ADHD. Efficacy is supported by a small double-blind placebo controlled crossover RCT (n=8) using clonidine (0.15–0.20 mg/day in three doses). Improvements were noted on teacher-rated ABC subscales for irritability, stereotypy, hyperactivity, and inappropriate speech ($P=0.01$; $P=0.05$; $P=0.03$; $P=0.05$, respectively) [23]. Teachers and parents both identified decreased appetite and drowsiness as significant adverse events in the treatment group.

Atypical antipsychotics

Using atypical antipsychotics to manage ADHD symptoms in ASD has been supported by analysis of secondary measures in RCTs of risperidone and aripiprazole targeting irritability [24–29]. Aripiprazole demonstrated statistically significant reduction in hyperactivity as rated on the ABC hyperactivity subscale relative to placebo controls (doses ranging from 5–15 mg/day) consistently in two RCTs [28,29]. Aman et al evaluated the impact of risperidone on attention using the Cancellation Task and identified no decline in the measures of attention and improvement in two areas of cognitive processing [30,31]. Nevertheless, atypical antipsychotic agents have a significant metabolic adverse event profile and their use should be guided carefully by evaluation of risk-to-benefit ratio.

Summary of evidence: treatment for attention deficit hyperactivity symptom cluster

Collectively, there is clear evidence to support the use of methylphenidate and, to some extent, atomoxetine, α2-agonists, and atypical antipsychotics as pharmacotherapy options for treating the ADHD symptom cluster in the context of ASD with moderate risk of adverse events. The response rates to these pharmacology agents are less than in non-ASD children and youth with similar profiles, and this should be explained to parents and youth when prescribing these medications. Further evidence is required to guide clinicians in matching appropriate patient phenotypic profiles to specific pharmacotherapies.

Irritability, aggression, and self-injurious behavior symptom cluster

Irritability, aggression, and self-injurious behaviors amongst children diagnosed with ASD are common. The etiology is variable and clinicians should evaluate for medical comorbidities (eg, GI disturbance, sleep difficulties), psychiatric illness, emotional regulation difficulties, communication/comprehension deficits, and difficulties in understanding the relationship between behaviors and consequences. Timely implementation of well-designed behavioral interventions may reduce the need for psychoactive medications, which are commonly employed for disruptive behavior in individuals with ASD [32]. However, the FDA has approved risperidone and aripiprazole for children with ASD and chronic irritability/impulsive aggression. Risperidone has also been approved by the European Medicines Agency (EMA) for this purpose.

Prior to newer antipsychotics, haloperidol was used with some success to mitigate aggression and improve global functioning in ASD, with evidence of a decrease in a variety of behaviors including tantrums, hyperactivity, withdrawal and stereotypies [33,34]. Haloperidol has fallen out of favor, however, due to the limiting factor of sedation and significant extrapyramidal adverse events; thus, haloperidol is not generally thought of as first-line management for maladaptive behaviors in autism.

Second generation antipsychotics have fewer and/or different, yet still significant, adverse events and are used as first-line management. This is supported by RCTs with aripiprazole (n=98–218 patients; aged 6–17 years) [28,29] and risperidone (n=79–101 patients, aged 5–17 years) [24,25,35]. Most studies used the ABC irritability subscale to assess irritability [19]. A meta-analysis showed that aripiprazole (combined n=308; 210 receiving aripiprazole) resulted in significant reduction in scores on the irritability (–6.17; $P<0.00001$), hyperactivity (–7.93; $P<0.00001$), and stereotypic behavior (–2.66; $P<0.00001$) subscales of the ABC when compared to placebo [36]. The response rate to aripiprazole varies from 52–56%, with a placebo response rate ranging from 14–35%. The positive response rate (as defined by a 25% reduction in the ABC irritability score and improvement on the Clinical Global Impression [CGI]-Improvement scale) to risperidone ranges from 64–69% vs. 12–31% in the placebo group. Somnolence, weight gain, and tremor were common adverse events reported in the treatment group.

A meta-analysis in 2007 reviewing three RCTs showed that risperidone leads to significant reduction in scores on the ABC irritability subscale (mean score on treatment of 8.09 lower than control [CI –12.99–3.19]) [37]. Risperidone was also associated with a significant increase in weight by 2.7 kg (95% CI; 1.15–2.41) vs. 1.0 kg in the placebo group over an 8-week period [37].

Mood stabilizers (primarily valproic acid, lamotrigine, and levetiracetam) have been evaluated for their ability to manage irritability and aggression in ASD. These agents are primarily used for their antiepileptic properties and their mechanisms of action are varied. Valproic acid/divalproex sodium is the most studied mood stabilizer in ASD. Two RCTs (n=27, ages 4–15 years; and n=30, ages 6–20 years, respectively) have yielded conflicting results [38,39]. In fact, Hellings et al reported no changes in the ABC irritability subscale [38]. However, this study was limited by high intra- and inter-participant variability in aggression frequency and severity, which impacts the power of the study. Interestingly, a large number of patients randomized to drug chose to stay on medication at the end of the trial.

Hollander et al used the CGI-Improvement scale and the ABC to assess irritability in response to divalproex [39]. A 62.5% positive response rate was noted in the divalproex group vs. 9.09% in the placebo group (Fischer's exact, $P=0.008$), with an odds ratio of 16.66. There was also a decrease in the ABC irritability subscale scores ($P=0.048$). Adverse events differentially affecting the valproate group included insomnia, skin rash, headache, and agitation. Effects on weight gain and uncommon effects on blood counts, liver function, pancreatic function, as well as hyperammonemic encephalopathy have been reported elsewhere. Lamotrigine and levetiracetam have shown no effect on irritability or global functioning in children with ASD [40,41]. Thus, the overall evidence for mood stabilizers in the management of irritability in ASD is equivocal.

Naltrexone, an opioid antagonist, also has some data to support potential efficacy for irritability and self-injury at an optimal dose of 1.0 mg/kg/day, based on small RCTs [42,43]. For example, Campbell et al (n=41 children) demonstrated a significant reduction in hyperactivity ($P=0.0002$) and a trend toward decreased self-injurious behavior that did not reach statistical significance [42]. Willemsen-Swinkels et al showed a reduction in hyperactivity ($P=0.003$) and irritability ($P=0.048$) based on scores on the ABC in 23 children treated with naltrexone 1 mg/kg [43].

A series of small, unreplicated trials have shown some benefit for a variety of additional compounds over placebo for the treatment of irritability in ASD. These include clonidine [23], methylphenidate [2], amantadine [44], clomipramine [45], pioglitazone [46], levocarnitine [47], and pentoxifyline [48], and this remains an area of active research.

Summary of evidence: treatment for irritability, aggression, self-injurious behavior symptom cluster

There is clear evidence to support the use of atypical antipsychotics risperidone and aripiprazole for the management of irritability and aggression in children and youth with ASD. This is limited, however, by significant weight gain and risk of drug-induced metabolic adverse events. Other atypicals often used for this purpose do not have adequate data to support their use yet. Evidence from mood stabilizers such as divalproex sodium and agents such as naltrexone suggests that they may decrease irritability in ASD but large clinical trials are needed.

Repetitive behaviors, obsessions, and compulsions symptom cluster

The core behavioral symptoms of ASD include restricted, repetitive patterns of behaviors, interests, or activities [1]. Repetitive behaviors in ASD tend to not be distressing on their own to the individual, although they may become distressing if interrupted. This behavior domain tends to be accompanied by general rigidity around rules and routines, producing distress around transitions or when flexibility is required. These behaviors differ from repetitive behaviors seen in obsessive compulsive disorder (OCD), which typically involve sequencing activities, checking, and ordering compulsions, and tend to be egodystonic. Still, at times it is difficult to differentiate repetitive behaviors that are specific to ASD versus OCD-like behaviors, especially in individuals with limited communication abilities.

Selective serotonin reuptake inhibitors

At least six RCTs have been conducted to evaluate the efficacy of selective serotonin reuptake inhibitors (SSRIs) on repetitive/stereotyped behaviors in ASD, although most have used small patient populations (n=12–149) [45,49–52]. An early study (n=12) evaluated the efficacy of clomipramine for treating repetitive stereotyped behaviors with a mean dose of 152mg per day, which showed a reduction in Modified Comprehensive Psychopathological Rating Scale OCD subscale (P=0.001) [49,53]. Remington et al evaluated the efficacy of clomipramine vs. haloperidol vs. placebo and found no changes on the ABC stereotypy subscale score for clomipramine [45]. Interestingly, only 37.5% of participants completed the clomipramine arm due to adverse events, whereas 69.7% and 65.6% completed the haloperidol and placebo arms, respectively.

A small RCT of fluoxetine in children with ASD showed some superiority over placebo [50]. However, the largest SSRI study (n=149) in ASD to date showed no effectiveness for citalopram in the management of repetitive behaviors [51].

A Cochrane review of SSRIs for repetitive behaviors in children with ASD suggested no benefit for this class of medications in this domain [54]. In the case of adults with ASD, there is some suggestion of efficacy for fluoxetine and fluvoxamine based on scores from the Yale-Brown Obsessive Compulsive Scale in two small RCTs [52,55,56]. Lastly, secondary analysis of the risperidone and aripiprazole trials have shown evidence of efficacy for reducing repetitive behaviors compared to placebo [7,57]. As noted above, the risk-to-benefit ratio should be examined every time such medications are prescribed to children and adolescents, especially for off-label use.

Anxiety and affective instability symptom cluster

Pharmacotherapy of anxiety in ASD is a very under-researched area. While there is evidence for using SSRIs, tricyclic antidepressants, and benzodiazepines for the management of anxiety in typically functioning children, there are no RCTs evaluating the efficacy of medications on symptoms of anxiety in ASD. Thus, clinicians need to use their own judgment when prescribing based on the evidence generated from children with anxiety and no neurodevelopmental impairments. Behavioral/cognitive-behavioral interventions remain the first-line of therapy to address anxiety in any child or youth.

Sleep problems

Sleep problems are present in up to 80% of children with ASD. Common reported challenges include circadian rhythm sleep disorders, parasomnias, insomnia, hypersomnia, sleep-related movement disorders, and abnormal objective sleep patterns. Melatonin has been the only medication evaluated via RCTs that has shown efficacy in reducing sleep-onset latency and decreasing night-time awakening. A systematic review identified that melatonin improves sleep duration by 73 minutes in the treatment group compared to 44 minutes with placebo, and increases sleep latency by 66 minutes (39 minutes for placebo) [58]. There was no impact on night-time awakenings [58].

Monitoring

It is important that clinicians monitor adverse events and metabolic complications that may occur with pharmacological agents used in the management of associated symptoms of ASD. Monitoring of stimulants and nonstimulants involves measurements of weight, height, heart rate, and blood pressure. α2-agonists can cause hypotension and monitoring of blood pressure is recommended. Antipsychotics can cause significant weight gain, extrapyramidal side effects, hyper/hypoprolactinemia, hyperlipidemia, and glucose abnormalities. Monitoring of weight, body mass index, lipid profile, fasting glucose level, prolactin levels, and evidence of extrapyramidal side effects using the AIMS [59] or a similar scale is advised (Table 5.1).

Pringsheim et al [60] provide an excellent review of evidence regarding the above recommendations, advising on second generation antipsychotics in children. Several bodies, such as the Autism Treatment Network and the Canadian Alliance for Monitoring Effectiveness and Safety of Antipsychotics in Childhood (CAMESA), have produced guidelines for such monitoring [61]. The Academy of Child and Adolescent Psychiatry (AACAP) has recently also published a practice parameter for assessment and treatment of children and adolescents with ASD, but do not include monitoring guidelines specific for this population [62].

Complementary and alternative medications

Although frequently used, evidence supporting the use of complementary and alternative medications is still lacking. For a review of complementary and alternative medicine treatment in ASD and a practical guide consider two reviews: [63,64]. The level of research available is variable and efficacy is not established for most complementary and alternative medicine treatments.

Symptom domain –Medication choice	Formulation	Dosing recommendations*	Baseline work-up	Adverse events	Monitoring	Clinical pearls
Hyperactivity/inattention						
–Methylphenidate	Oral solution: 1 mg/mL Tablet: 5 mg,10 mg, 15 mg SR: 10–20 mg LA: 10–40 mg Osmotic CR: 18–54 mg CR: 10–50 mg	**Immediate-release:** Starting dose: 2.5 –5 mg BID Increase by: 2.5–5 mg/24 hr weekly Dose range: 5.0–60 mg/day OR 0.25–1.0 mg/kg/day (divided doses) Maximum dose: 2 mg/kg/24 hr or 60 mg/24 hr **Extended-release:** Starting dose: 10–20 mg po QAM Increase by: 10–20 mg weekly Maximum dose: 60 mg/day	**Consider:** ECG and cardiac consult if there is a family history of cardiac illness and subject has an underline cardiac pathology Baseline HR, BP, weight, height, BMI	**CNS:** Irritability Decreased appetite Difficulty falling asleep Emotional outburst Social withdrawal Drowsiness **GIT:** Abdominal pain Nausea/vomiting Nausea Dry Mouth **CVS:** Tachycardia Palpitation Hypotension Hypertension	**Must track:** Weight Height BP BMI **Consider:** CBC if subject has pallor on examination due to risk of nutrition-based anemia	Contraindicated in children with structural abnormalities, MAOI use There is initial growth delay (weight and height) but will normalize over time Not indicated in children <5 years May lower seizure threshold Consider psychiatric disorders if psychosis precipitated with use Tics may/may not be exacerbated

Table 5.1 *(continues opposite)*.

Symptom domain – Medication choice	Formulation	Dosing recommendations*	Baseline work-up	Adverse events	Monitoring	Clinical pearls
Hyperactivity/inattention						
- Atomoxetine	**Capsules:** 10 mg, 18 mg, 25 mg, 40 mg, 60 mg	**Children <70 kg:** Starting dose: 0.5 mg/kg/day Increase to 0.8 mg/kg/day then up to 1.2 mg/kg/day ÷ OD or BID Maximum dose: 1.4 mg/kg/day or 100 mg/day, whichever is less **Children >70kg:** Starting dose: 40 mg/day Increase to: 60 mg/day then up to 80 mg/day ÷OD or BID Maximum dose: 100 mg/day ÷ OD or BID Increase in doses can occur minimum 3–10 day intervals	**Consider:** Baseline HR, BP	**CNS:** Fatigue Difficulty falling asleep Emotional lability **GIT:** Decreased appetite Nausea/vomiting Nausea Weight loss **CVS:** Tachycardia Rhinitis	**Must track:** HR BP	Atomoxetine may take 4-7 weeks before therapeutic effects are seen Should discontinue any MAOI agents before starting Evidence supporting impact on hyperactivity and inattention Some anti-anxiety properties (mild)

Table 5.1 (*continues overleaf*).

Symptom domain –Medication choice	Formulation	Dosing recommendations*	Baseline work-up	Adverse events	Monitoring	Clinical pearls
Hyperactivity/inattention						
–Clonidine	**Tablet:** 0.1 mg, 0.2 mg, 0.3 mg	Starting dose: 0.05 mg/day QHS Increase by 0.05 mg/day every 3–7 days Maximum dose: 0.4 mg/day Titrated dosing should be divided as TID-QID For extended release: Starting dose 0.1 mg QHS Increase by 0.1 mg (bid dosing) Maximum dose: 0.4 mg/day	**Consider:** Baseline HR, BP	**CNS:** Sedation **CVS:** Hypotension	**Must track:** HR BP	Evidence supporting impact on hyperactivity Evidence to support some impact on irritability Some anti-anxiety properties (dosing at 0.15–0.5 mg/day) Rebound hypertension with discontinuation or with only OD dosing
–Guanfacine XR	**Tablet:** 1 mg, 2 mg, 3 mg, 4 mg	Starting dose: 1 mg/day OD Increase by: 1 mg/week Maximum dose: 4 mg/day OD	**Consider:** Baseline HR, BP	**CNS:** Sedation Fatigue Insomnia **CVS:** Hypotension Bradycardia Syncope	**Must track:** HR BP	Evidence supporting impact on hyperactivity Evidence to support some impact on irritability Precaution in hepatic or renal failure

Table 5.1 *(continues opposite).*

Symptom domain – Medication choice	Formulation	Dosing recommendations*	Baseline work-up	Adverse events	Monitoring	Clinical pearls
Irritability/aggression						
– Aripiprazole	**Tablet:** 2 mg, 5 mg, 10 mg, 15 mg, 20 mg, 30 mg	Starting dose: 2 mg/day OD Increase by: 2–5 mg every week Maximum dose: 15 mg/day OD (average dose in autism trials:5.0–7.5 mg/day)	**Consider:** ECG Ascertain family history risk for diabetes mellitus, hyperlipidemia and cardiac pathology Bloods; Fasting glucose, HbA1c, lipid profile, liver enzymes, prolactin level Baseline HR, BP, weight, height, BMI, waist circumference Baseline evaluation of evidence of extra pyramidal side effects	**Metabolic:** Hyperlipidemia Diabetes mellitus Weight gain Hyperglycemia **Other:** Orthostatic Hypotension Drowsiness Extrapyramidal side effects	Monitor risk benefit ratio at each visit Blood work every 3–6 months for the first year Monitor for extrapyramidal side effects at all visits Monitor weight, BMI, BP at each visit	Can lower seizure threshold Nausea can occur at lower doses and may improve with dose increase Weight gain noted up to 2 kg in 2 months Low prolactin levels noted, its significance is not yet established

Table 5.1 (*continues overleaf*).

Symptom domain – Medication choice	Formulation	Dosing recommendations*	Baseline work-up	Adverse events	Monitoring	Clinical pearls
Irritability/aggression						
– Risperidone	**Oral solution:** 1 mg/ml Tablet: 0.25 mg, 0.5 mg, 1 mg, 2 mg, 3 mg, 4 mg, 5 mg	Starting dose: 0.25 mg/day given OD or BID Increase by: 0.5–1.0 mg every week Maximum dose: 3.5 mg/day in children and up to 4 mg/day in adolescents	Same as aripiprazole	Same as aripiprazole	Same as aripiprazole	Significant weight gain associated with risperidone up to 2.7 kg in 2 months Elevated prolactin levels noted
Sleep						
– Melatonin	Over the counter, multiple preparations	Starting dose: 2 mg/day given at night Increase by: 2–3 mg as needed Maximum dose: up to 10 mg reported in studies, no consensus on maximum dose noted.	None indicated	**Rare:** Abdominal cramps Fatigue Headache Irritability	Review sleep history and sleep hygiene techniques if no response noted	Ensure sleep routine is in place Rule out an organic cause for sleep problems (eg, sleep apnea) Ensure room is quiet, dark to help with initiating sleep

Table 5.1 (*continued***)** Medication dosing and monitoring recommendation for use in autism spectrum disorder (ASD) for pediatric patients, based on symptom-based approach. *dose range reflects typical dosing within the pediatric population. BID, twice daily; BMI, body mass index; BP, blood pressure; CBC, complete blood count; CNS, central nervous system; CR, controlled release; CVS, cardiovascular system; ECG, electrocardiogram; FR, fast-release; GIT, gastrointestinal tract; HbA1c, glycated hemoglobin; HR, heart rate; LA, long-acting; MAOI, monoamine oxidase inhibitors; OD once-daily; SR, slow-release; TID, thrice-daily; XR, extended-release; QAM, every day before noon; QHS, every night at bedtime; QID, four times daily.

Conclusions

Given the lack of translation of basic science findings into molecular targets for drug development at this time, medications are used to treat associated symptoms of ASD in an effort to remove barriers and facilitate learning that is provided through conventional teaching settings such as school, or from behavioral and/or psychosocial interventions. Careful monitoring of all medications is necessary as per available guidelines. With the explosion of genomic findings and data from systems neuroscience, a series of molecular targets present themselves and several clinical trials are currently underway with the aim of addressing core symptom domains in ASD for the first time. Still, given that ASD is a neurodevelopmental disorder of skill acquisition (and maintenance), existing and future medication management will always need to be paired with effective educational, behavioral, and/or psychosocial interventions so that they can facilitate skill acquisition.

References

1 American Psychiatric Association. *Diagnostic and Statistical Manual of Mental Disorders.* 5th edn. Washington, D.C.: American Psychiatric Association; 2013.

2 Quintana H, Birmaher B, Stedge D, et al. Use of methylphenidate in the treatment of children with autistic disorder. *J Autism Dev Disord.* 1995;25:283-294.

3 Handen BL, Johnson CR, Lubetsky M. Efficacy of methylphenidate among children with autism and symptoms of attention-deficit hyperactivity disorder. *J Autism Dev Disord.* 2000;30:245-255.

4 Research Units on Pediatric Psychopharmacology Autism Network. Randomized, controlled, crossover trial of methylphenidate in pervasive developmental disorders with hyperactivity. *Arch Gen Psychiatry.* 2005;62:1266-1274.

5 Posey DJ, Aman MG, McCracken JT, et al. Positive effects of methylphenidate on inattention and hyperactivity in pervasive developmental disorders: an analysis of secondary measures. *Biological Psychiatry.* 2007;61:538-544.

6 Ghuman JK, Aman MG, Lecavalier L, et al. Randomized, placebo-controlled, crossover study of methylphenidate for attention-deficit/hyperactivity disorder symptoms in preschoolers with developmental disorders. *J Child Adolesc Psychopharmacol.* 2009;19:329-339.

7 Pearson DA, Santos CW, Aman MG, et al. Effects of extended release methylphenidate treatment on ratings of attention-deficit/hyperactivity disorder (ADHD) and associated behavior in children with autism spectrum disorders and ADHD symptoms. *J Child Adolesc Psychopharmacol.* 2013;23:337-351.

8 Reichow B, Volkmar FR, Bloch MH. Systematic review and meta-analysis of pharmacological treatment of the symptoms of attention-deficit/hyperactivity disorder in children with pervasive developmental disorders. *J Autism Dev Disord.* 2013;43:2435-2441.

9 Conners CK, Sitarenios G, Parker JD, Epstein JN. The Revised Conners' Parent Rating Scale (CPRS-R): factor structure, reliability, and criterion validity. *J Abnorm Child Psychol.* 1998;26:257-268.

10 Bussing R, Fernandez M, Harwood M, et al. Parent and teacher SNAP-IV ratings of attention deficit hyperactivity disorder symptoms: psychometric properties and normative ratings from a school district sample. *Assessment.* 2008;15:317-28.

11 Conners CK, Sitarenios G, Parker JD, Epstein JN. Revision and restandardization of the Conners' Teacher Rating Scale (CTRS-R): factor structure, reliability, and criterion validity. *J Abnorm Child* Psychol. 1998;26:279-291.

12 Aman MG, Buican B, Arnold LE. Methylphenidate treatment in children with borderline IQ and mental retardation: analysis of three aggregated studies. *J Child Adolesc Psychopharmacol.* 2003;13:29-40.

13 Elia J, Borcherding BG, Rapoport JL, Keysor CS. Methylphenidate and dextroamphetamine treatments of hyperactivity: are there true nonresponders? *Psychiatry Research.* 1991;6:141-155.

14 Campbell M, Small AM, Collins PJ, Friedman E, David R, Genieser N. Levodopa and levoamphetamine: A crossover study in young schizophrenic children. *Curr Ther Res Clin Exp.* 1976;19:70-86.

15 Busner J, Targum SD, Miller DS. The Clinical Global Impressions scale: errors in understanding and use. *Compr Psychiatry.* 2009;50:257-262.

16 Mahajan R, Bernal MP, Panzer R, et al. Clinical practice pathways for evaluation and medication choice for attention-deficit/hyperactivity disorder symptoms in autism spectrum disorders. *Pediatrics.* 2012; 130(Suppl 2):S125-S138.

17 Arnold LE, Aman MG, Cook AM, et al. Atomoxetine for hyperactivity in autism spectrum disorders: placebo-controlled crossover pilot trial. *J Am Acad Child Adolesc Psychiatry.* 2006; 45:1196-1205.

18 Harfterkamp M, van de Loo-Neus G, Minderaa RB, et al. A randomized double-blind study of atomoxetine versus placebo for attention-deficit/hyperactivity disorder symptoms in children with autism spectrum disorder. *J Am Acad Child Adolesc Psychiatry.* 2012;51:733-741.

19 Aman MG, Singh NN, Stewart AW, Field CJ. The aberrant behavior checklist: a behavior rating scale for the assessment of treatment effects. *Am J Ment Defic.* 1985;89:485-491.

20 Zhang S, Faries DE, Vowles M, Michelson D. ADHD Rating Scale IV: psychometric properties from a multinational study as a clinician-administered instrument. *Int J Methods Psychiatr Res.* 2005;14:186-201.

21 Kelsey DK, Sumner CR, Casat CD, et al. Once-daily atomoxetine treatment for children with attention-deficit/hyperactivity disorder, including an assessment of evening and morning behavior: a double-blind, placebo-controlled trial. *Pediatrics.* 2004;114:e1-e8.

22 Handen BL, Sahl R, Hardan AY. Guanfacine in children with autism and/or intellectual disabilities. *J Dev Behav Pediatr.* 2008;29:303-308.

23 Jaselskis CA, Cook EH, Jr., Fletcher KE, Leventhal BL. Clonidine treatment of hyperactive and impulsive children with autistic disorder. *J Clin Psychopharmacol.* 1992;12:322-327.

24 McCracken JT, McGough J, Shah B, et al. Risperidone in children with autism and serious behavioral problems. *N Engl J Med.* 2002;347:314-321.

25 Shea S, Turgay A, Carroll A, et al. Risperidone in the treatment of disruptive behavioral symptoms in children with autistic and other pervasive developmental disorders. *Pediatrics.* 2004;114:e634-e641.

26 Nagaraj R, Singhi P, Malhi P. Risperidone in children with autism: randomized, placebo-controlled, double-blind study. *J Child Neurol.* 2006;21:450-455.

27 Pandina GJ, Bossie CA, Youssef E, Zhu Y, Dunbar F. Risperidone improves behavioral symptoms in children with autism in a randomized, double-blind, placebo-controlled trial. *J Autism Dev Disord.* 2007;37:367-373.

28 Owen R, Sikich L, Marcus RN, et al. Aripiprazole in the treatment of irritability in children and adolescents with autistic disorder. *Pediatrics.* 2009;124:1533-1540.

29 Marcus RN, Owen R, Kamen L, et al. A placebo-controlled, fixed-dose study of aripiprazole in children and adolescents with irritability associated with autistic disorder. *J Am Acad Child Adolesc Psychiatry.* 2009;48:1110-1119.

30 Aman MG, Hollway JA, McDougle CJ, et al. Cognitive effects of risperidone in children with autism and irritable behavior. *J Child Adolesc Psychopharmacol.* 2008;18:227-236.

31 Barkley RA. The ecological validity of laboratory and analogue assessment methods of ADHD symptoms. *J Abnorm Child Psychol.* 1991;19:149-178.

32 Sharma A, Shaw SR. Efficacy of risperidone in managing maladaptive behaviors for children with autistic spectrum disorder: a meta-analysis. *J Pediatr Health Care.* 2012;26:291-299.

33 Anderson LT, Campbell M, Grega DM, Perry R, Small AM, Green WH. Haloperidol in the treatment of infantile autism: effects on learning and behavioral symptoms. *Am J Psychiatry.* 1984;141:1195-202.

34 Anderson LT, Campbell M, Adams P, Small AM, Perry R, Shell J. The effects of haloperidol on discrimination learning and behavioral symptoms in autistic children. *J Autism Dev Disord.* 1989;19:227-239.

35 McDougle CJ, Scahill L, Aman MG, et al. Risperidone for the core symptom domains of autism: results from the study by the autism network of the research units on pediatric psychopharmacology. *Am J Psychiatry.* 2005;162:1142-1148.

36 Ching H, Pringsheim T. Aripiprazole for autism spectrum disorders (ASD). *Cochrane Database of Syst Rev.* 2012(5):CD009043.

37 Jesner OS, Aref-Adib M, Coren E. Risperidone for autism spectrum disorder. *Cochrane Database of Syst Rev.* 2007(1):CD005040.

38 Hellings JA, Weckbaugh M, Nickel EJ, et al. A double-blind, placebo-controlled study of valproate for aggression in youth with pervasive developmental disorders. *J Child Adolesc Psychopharmacol.* 2005;15:682-692.

39 Hollander E, Chaplin W, Soorya L, et al. Divalproex sodium vs placebo for the treatment of irritability in children and adolescents with autism spectrum disorders. *Neuropsychopharmacology.* 2010;35:990-998.

40 Belsito KM, Law PA, Kirk KS, Landa RJ, Zimmerman AW. Lamotrigine therapy for autistic disorder: a randomized, double-blind, placebo-controlled trial. *J Autism Dev Disord.* 2001;31:175-181.

41 Wasserman S, Iyengar R, Chaplin WF, et al. Levetiracetam versus placebo in childhood and adolescent autism: a double-blind placebo-controlled study. *Int Clin Psychopharmacol.* 2006;21:363-367.

42 Campbell M, Anderson LT, Small AM, Adams P, Gonzalez NM, Ernst M. Naltrexone in autistic children: behavioral symptoms and attentional learning. *J Am Acad Child Adolesc Psychiatry.* 1993;32:1283-1291.

43 Willemsen-Swinkels SH, Buitelaar JK, Weijnen FG, van Engeland H. Placebo-controlled acute dosage naltrexone study in young autistic children. *Psychiatry Res.* 1995;58:203-215.

44 King BH, Wright DM, Handen BL, et al. Double-blind, placebo-controlled study of amantadine hydrochloride in the treatment of children with autistic disorder. *J Am Acad Child Adolesc Psychiatry.* 2001;40:658-665.

45 Remington G, Sloman L, Konstantareas M, Parker K, Gow R. Clomipramine versus haloperidol in the treatment of autistic disorder: a double-blind, placebo-controlled, crossover study. *J Clin Psychopharmacol.* 2001;21:440-444.

46 Boris M, Kaiser CC, Goldblatt A, et al. Effect of pioglitazone treatment on behavioral symptoms in autistic children. *J Neuroinflammation.* 2007;4:3.

47 Geier DA, Kern JK, Davis G, et al. A prospective double-blind, randomized clinical trial of levocarnitine to treat autism spectrum disorders. *Med Sci Monit.* 2011;17:PI15-PI23.

48 Akhondzadeh S, Fallah J, Mohammadi MR, et al. Double-blind placebo-controlled trial of pentoxifylline added to risperidone: effects on aberrant behavior in children with autism. *Prog Neuropsychopharmacol Biol Psychiatry.* 2010;34:32-36.

49 Gordon CT, State RC, Nelson JE, Hamburger SD, Rapoport JL. A double-blind comparison of clomipramine, desipramine, and placebo in the treatment of autistic disorder. *Arch Gen Psychiatry.* 1993;50:441-447.

50 Hollander E, Phillips A, Chaplin W, et al. A placebo controlled crossover trial of liquid fluoxetine on repetitive behaviors in childhood and adolescent autism. *Neuropsychopharmacology.* 2005;30:582-589.

51 King BH, Hollander E, Sikich L, et al. Lack of efficacy of citalopram in children with autism spectrum disorders and high levels of repetitive behavior: citalopram ineffective in children with autism. *Arch Gen Psychiatry.* 2009;66:583-590.

52 McDougle CJ, Naylor ST, Cohen DJ, Volkmar FR, Heninger GR, Price LH. A double-blind, placebo-controlled study of fluvoxamine in adults with autistic disorder. *Arch Gen Psychiatry.* 1996;53:1001-1008.

53 Asberg M, Montgomery SA, Perris C, Schalling D, Sedvall G. A comprehensive psychopathological rating scale. *Acta Psychiatrica Scandinavica Supplementum.* 1978:5-27.

54 Williams K, Brignell A, Randall M, Silove N, Hazell P. Selective serotonin reuptake inhibitors (SSRIs) for autism spectrum disorders (ASD). *Cochrane Database Syst Rev.* 2013;8:CD004677.

55 Scahill L, Riddle MA, McSwiggin-Hardin M, et al. Children's Yale-Brown Obsessive Compulsive Scale: reliability and validity. *J Am Acad Child Adolesc Psychiatry.* 1997;36:844-852.

56 Hollander E, Soorya L, Chaplin W, et al. A double-blind placebo-controlled trial of fluoxetine for repetitive behaviors and global severity in adult autism spectrum disorders. *Am J Psychiatry.* 2012;169:292-299.

57 Aman MG, Kasper W, Manos G, et al. Line-item analysis of the Aberrant Behavior Checklist: results from two studies of aripiprazole in the treatment of irritability associated with autistic disorder. *J Child Adolesc Psychopharmacol.* 2010;20:415-422.

58 Rossignol DA, Frye RE. Melatonin in autism spectrum disorders: a systematic review and meta-analysis. *Dev Med Child Neurol.* 2011;53:783-792.

59 Rey JM, Hunt GE, Johnson GF. Assessment of tardive dyskinesia in psychiatric outpatients using a standardized rating scale. *Aust N Z J Psychiatry.* 1981;15:33-37.

60 Pringsheim T, Panagiotopoulos C, Davidson J, Ho J. Evidence-based recommendations for monitoring safety of second-generation antipsychotics in children and youth. *Paediatr Child Health (Oxford).* 2011;16:581-589.

61 Canadian Alliance for Monitoring Effectiveness and Safety of Antipsychotics in Children. (CAMESA). How to monitor antipsychotic drug safety. http://camesaguideline.org. Accessed January 4, 2015.

62 Volkmar F, Siegel M, Woodbury-Smith M, King B, McCracken J, State M. Practice parameter for the assessment and treatment of children and adolescents with autism spectrum disorder. *J Am Acad Child Adolesc Psychiatry.* 2014;53:237-257.

63 Huffman LC, Sutcliffe TL, Tanner IS, Feldman HM. Management of symptoms in children with autism spectrum disorders: a comprehensive review of pharmacologic and complementary-alternative medicine treatments. Journal of developmental and behavioral pediatrics. *J Dev Behav Pediatr.* 2011;32:56-68.

64 Akins RS, Angkustsiri K, Hansen RL. Complementary and alternative medicine in autism: an evidence-based approach to negotiating safe and efficacious interventions with families. *Neurotherapeutics.* 2010;7:307-319.

Chapter 6

Behavioral and educational interventions

Isabel M Smith, Susan E Bryson

Key Learning Objectives

By the end of this chapter, readers will be able to identify:

- elements of evidence-based approaches to early intervention;
- important considerations for managing maladaptive behavior;
- key elements of effective social skills interventions;
- considerations relevant to academic programs for children, youth and young adults with autism spectrum disorder (ASD); and
- service needs for adults with ASD.

Following a diagnosis of ASD, parents understandably seek recommendations about treatment for their child. Advice regarding intervention will depend on the age and presentation of the individual; in particular, his/her developmental level and the severity of ASD symptoms. Globally, the goals of behavioral and educational interventions for individuals with ASD are to:

- facilitate learning and acquisition of skills that meet individual and family needs;
- eliminate or reduce behavior that may interfere with such learning; and
- enhance quality of life for all family members.

The heterogeneous presentation of ASD becomes more salient with age. This is at least in part because those diagnosed youngest tend to be among

E. Anagnostou and J. Brian (eds.), *Clinician's Manual on Autism Spectrum Disorder*, DOI 10.1007/978-3-319-03056-2_6

the most severely affected; hence, similar intervention targets and methods may be appropriate very early in development. For example, a program serving toddlers with ASD likely will have the acquisition of effective language/communication skills as a central target of intervention. In contrast, by the early school years, diagnosed children will range from those with significant intellectual disability and limited communication skills to children who are highly verbal but socially and behaviorally atypical, with treatment needs varying accordingly.

Behavioral interventions

In general, interventions found to be effective in ASD are based on the empirically-derived principles of learning [1]. The field of applied behavior analysis (ABA) is dedicated to the application of strategies based on learning principles to address problems in human behavior [2]. ABA delineates procedures that either increase or decrease behavior, in the case of desirable (adaptive) or interfering (maladaptive) forms of behavior, respectively. The three-term contingency (antecedent-behavior-consequence [A-B-C]) is a fundamental construct in ABA, and manipulations of this contingency (eg, use of reinforcing consequences, which produce increases in the preceding behavior) form the basis of ABA procedures. ABA-based teaching strategies vary in how readily they can be implemented without extensive technical expertise and the context in which they can be carried out.

As an extreme example, discrete trial teaching (DTT) involves many repetitions of precisely defined A-B-C sequences ("massed trials") and is typically conducted in controlled settings (eg, a quiet room with only the child and therapist present). In contrast, "naturalistic" ABA-based procedures capitalize on opportunities for teaching that are present in daily activities in typical environments such as the home, preschool, or school [3]. Some evidence supports both approaches; the critical but not yet adequately addressed question is which ABA procedures are best suited for which specific forms of behavior in which contexts, and for which individuals [1,3]. One important challenge in this field is that much of the high-quality evidence is derived from single-subject design studies. This research design has established the efficacy of many component

ABA-based procedures used to address behavioral deficits and excesses, including those associated with ASD [4]. However, further research is needed testing the overall efficacy of programs that combine these procedures, as well as the effectiveness of service delivery models that implement treatment at the community level.

Early intervention

As an example, in most jurisdictions in North America, specialized early intervention programs are available for preschoolers diagnosed with ASD. Intervention programs for young children with ASD are often characterized as either comprehensive (multiple developmental domains are addressed within the program), or specific (targets of treatment are more focused) [3]. Many comprehensive programs are variants of the model developed at the University of California at Los Angeles (UCLA) by Lovaas, a pioneer in the use of behavioral methods to treat ASD [5]. These early intensive behavioural intervention (EIBI) programs may be referred to as based on the "UCLA", "Lovaas", or "Young Autism Project" model [6]. These are often erroneously called "ABA programs". (Note that, as described above, ABA refers to a scientific discipline rather than to any specific intervention model and is not ASD-specific).

Numerous systematic reviews and meta-analyses have concluded that EIBI programs based on the UCLA model yield improvements in cognitive, language, and adaptive functioning for many children with ASD (see [7,8] for a recent overview of meta-analyses and Cochrane review). The factor associated with the best outcomes for children appears to be the quality of EIBI, as evidenced by expert supervision and formal monitoring of fidelity to the treatment procedures [7]. However, although this is the best available information, the quality of the evidence is low when evaluated against rigorous standards [8]. The inherent difficulties in conducting randomized controlled trials (RCTs) of such complex and long-term (2-to-4-year RCTs) means that few well-controlled efficacy trials exist [9]. Other limited evidence on the effectiveness of early intervention programs for preschoolers with ASD comes from community-based programs. For example, data from Canada and Sweden suggest that children's outcomes can be enhanced through wide-scale implementation of well supervised ABA-based intervention programs [10–14].

Only one study has compared the efficacy of three high-quality preschool programs for children with ASD, which involved comparing two well-known intervention programs (Treatment and Education for Autistic and Communication Handicapped [TEACCH] and Learning Experiences and Alternative Program for Preschoolers and their Parents [LEAP]) with a control program that did not espouse a specific treatment model [15]. Each program combined elements, including behavioral strategies (eg, reinforcement of desirable behavior) and other components. For example, the TEACCH program entails considerable emphasis on organizing the child's environment to provide concrete cues to appropriate behavior (eg, providing designated locations for tasks-to-be-completed and for finished activities, comparable to 'in' and 'out' boxes). Children enrolled in all three programs showed improvements in multiple areas of functioning after one year of treatment; there were no significant differences in outcomes across programs [15]. These results suggest that elements common to high-quality programs for preschoolers with ASD may be more critical than the specific aspects that differentiate them (Table 6.1).

As the age of diagnosis of ASD has decreased, a corresponding need has become evident for forms of intervention tailored to the needs of toddlers. One such program, the Early Start Denver Model (ESDM), has been shown to produce marked improvements in children's communication and other skills [16]. The ESDM incorporates naturalistic ABA-based strategies within a developmental framework and has the virtue of being manualized and therefore accessible to a wide range of potential users [17].

Parent education and training

One component that is common to effective early interventions for ASD is the involvement of parents [18]. In some EIBI models, this involvement may entail parents acting as therapists in structured DTT sessions [19]. Other treatment models promote parents' use of naturalistic ABA-based methods such as Pivotal Response Treatment which can be readily learned by parents and incorporated into everyday routines [20–22]. Children's ability to use skills across contexts (ie, generalization) is maximized by

Qualifications and supervision of staff	In addition to formal early childhood development and/or special education qualifications, experience working with children with ASD with similar characteristics is important. A high staff:child ratio allows individualized attention to the needs of the child with ASD.
Environment	A calm, organized physical environment with opportunities for individual, small group, and large group play.
Program content/targets of intervention	A program that addresses the key needs of young children with ASD by placing emphasis on functional communication and language skills, facilitating social interaction, and the development of daily living skills. The program should have well-articulated procedures for supporting skill acquisition and managing behavior problems.
Intervention methods; monitoring of fidelity of treatment	A program that utilizes systematic teaching by using established behavioral principles and other evidence-based strategies to address developmentally appropriate goals.
Intensity of intervention	A program that engages children in planned activities for a substantial proportion of waking hours, whether in one-on-one therapy, structured group activities within a daycare or preschool, and/or giving parents the skills to teach their children in the context of daily routines at home.

Table 6.1 Key considerations for choosing an intervention program for a preschooler with an autism spectrum disorder. ASD, autism spectrum disorder.

the use of naturalistic interventions and parent training, which combine to enable children to practice skills throughout daily life [23].

Parent training can be accomplished in group format [24] or via individual coaching [25]. A 2013 meta-analysis demonstrated that parent-mediated interventions may yield improved parent-child interactions, as well as an increase children's language skills and a decrease in the severity of ASD symptoms [26]. However, this literature is affected by methodological and analytic weaknesses. Moreover, the efficacy of the strategies that are taught to parents, and the fidelity with which these strategies are implemented by parents, determine whether they improve functioning. For example, an RCT evaluating a widely implemented parent-mediated program that was designed to enhance communication abilities of children with ASD produced no significant overall gains in children's communication skills, nor in parent responsiveness [27]. Whether these results are due to limitations in the techniques themselves or in parents' ability to use them effectively is a matter for further research. However, some parent programs targeting children's communication may offer indirect benefits, such as improving preschoolers' early social-communicative behavior with parents (eg, initiating interactions, sharing attention) [28].

Among older (school-aged) children with ASD, parental training in behavioral methods can be effective both in promoting positive behavior and managing disruptive behavior [29–31]. In children with ASD who developed severely disruptive behavior problems, reductions in noncompliance and irritability were observed when parents were enrolled in a 3-month manualized behavioral program [32]. In an RCT, the same behavioral program produced some additional benefit when evaluated as an adjunct to a pharmacological intervention (ie, risperidone) [33].

Interventions for disruptive behavioral problems

As a consequence of their limited communication skills and difficulties with behavioral flexibility (eg, coping with change or the unexpected), as well as high anxiety and possibly atypical reactions to sensory experiences, individuals with ASD are at increased risk for displaying disruptive behavior problems [18]. These may be manifested as tantrums, aggression, property destruction or self-injurious behavior.

Positive behavior (interventions) and support (PBS/PBIS) [34] is an approach to addressing behavior problems that emphasizes not only consequences for undesirable behavior ("C" in the A-B-C contingency) but also antecedents ("A"). That is, a major focus of PBIS is teaching skills to individuals and engineering their environments so as to prevent the circumstances that precipitate problematic behavior. The process of determining the antecedent conditions associated with the behavior problem (and the reinforcing consequences) is called functional behavioral assessment or functional analysis [35]. For example, a child may learn to engage in self-injurious behavior such as banging her head on her desk because adults reliably remove the requirement to comply with a difficult task. On the other hand, head or earache pain might be associated with such behavior. Understanding the *function* of the behavior permits a tailored approach to correcting the problem (eg, teaching skills required to master a task; treating a physical problem; Table 6.2). Timely implementation of well-designed behavioral interventions may reduce the

- Rule out underlying medical causes for problem behavior (eg, ear or dental pain).
- Look for patterns in order to identify its function(s) (when, where, with whom does the behavior typically occur? What happens immediately before and after the behavior?).
- Consider consultation with a professional who is trained in behavior analysis and development of behavioral intervention programs (eg, Board Certified Behavior Analyst; some specialized psychologists; some special educators).

Table 6.2 Key considerations for managing behavior problems in individuals with autism spectrum disorder.

need for psychoactive medications, which are commonly employed for disruptive behavior in individuals with ASD (see Chapter 5).

Social skills interventions

One of the most pressing areas of need for all individuals with ASD is the enhancement of the ability to engage in flexible and satisfying social interactions, especially with peers. Group social skills interventions are often offered to children and youth with ASD, especially those who are more intellectually able. There is some evidence to support this practice. A meta-analysis of five RCTs demonstrated positive effects on overall social competence, and to a lesser extent, quality of life measures [36]. Transfer of learned skills to contexts outside the social skills training group is a major challenge for individuals with ASD. Therefore, it is critical that social skills programs explicitly address generalization to everyday settings. A meta-analysis of 115 studies of social skills interventions that used single-case research methods (rather than RCT designs), involving 343 participants with ASD, similarly suggested benefit [37]. Many studies reviewed did not specify treatment parameters sufficiently well to allow recommendation of any particular approach. However, recent data on the Program for the Education and Enrichment of Relational Skills (PEERS) indicate that the social skills of school-aged children [38], adolescents [39], and young adults [40] with ASD can be improved with participation in this manualized parent- /caregiver-assisted program [41,42].

Another promising avenue for teaching social (and other) skills is to engage typically developing same-aged children/youth as intervention agents for their peers with ASD. Such peer-mediated interventions have shown positive effects. A meta-analysis of 45 studies conducted using single-subject research methods indicated that peer-mediated approaches produced positive outcomes for a range of targets, including social interactions [43]. Typically developing school-aged children can not only serve as positive role models for children with ASD, but can be taught to use simple strategies during enjoyable play activities to elicit more appropriate social behavior from their peers with ASD (Table 6.3). Indeed, an RCT has demonstrated the superiority of a peer-mediated social skills intervention over an alternative program in which children with ASD in Grades 1–5 received direct instruction from an adult [44].

• Involvement of peers is important but systematic teaching of specific skills, rather than mere exposure to peers, is necessary for learning social skills.
• Social skills are best developed with peers and during preferred activities.

Table 6.3 Key considerations for social skills programs for children with autism spectrum disorder.

Educational interventions

It is important to ensure that both academic and non-academic goals are incorporated into individual educational plans (IEPs) or individual program plans (IPPs) for children with ASD. These plans may resemble programming for preschoolers with ASD, particularly among the more severely affected. However, other more able children with ASD will be served within inclusive settings with relatively minor modifications to the regular curriculum. Contrary to some claims, no specific profile of cognitive skills is associated with ASD. Although a pattern of lower verbal cognitive skills relative to nonverbal performance skills is common, this 'nonverbal advantage' is by no means universal. Indeed, other individuals with ASD may show the opposite pattern; that is, relatively stronger verbal abilities [45]. Yet others may show no significant discrepancies between verbal and nonverbal abilities. Other aspects of cognition are also variable in ASD; slow processing and problems with executive functions (eg, attentional control, working memory) are common [46] but vary in severity.

The prevalence of intellectual disability (ID) in ASD has been a moving target as the definition of ASD has evolved in recent decades. However, a recent estimate is that about 40% of children with ASD demonstrate comorbid intellectual disability [47]. Many individuals with ASD but without ID meet criteria for a specific learning disability (eg, in reading or math). The newly revised Diagnostic and Statistical Manual of Mental

Disorders, 5th edition (DSM-5) [48] provides a framework for formal recognition of these characteristics by directing diagnosticians to specify the additional disorders/disabilities that may accompany ASD.

Given these considerations regarding intellectual abilities, academic programming should follow from the individual profile (ie, cognitive and academic strengths and weaknesses) defined in a formal neuropsychological/psychoeducational assessment. To optimize self-esteem and emotional well-being, academic programming should focus on developing the student's strengths and interests rather than focussing exclusively on the remediation of deficits. Other basic educational principles are related to the need to adjust teaching methods to accommodate characteristics associated with ASD such as difficulty with generalization, especially as it pertains to application of knowledge in real world situations. That is, for many skills, explicit teaching in the context in which the skill must be used is necessary for the individual to demonstrate competence.

In some jurisdictions, specialized academic programs, classrooms, or even schools are available to meet the needs of children and youth with ASD. Ideally, educational programs for children and youth with ASD will address social and adaptive behavior needs (including those related to 'street-proofing' and personal safety), as well as academic subjects. Guidelines for educational best practices that address all of these areas are available from two recent major initiatives in the US [3,49]. Unfortunately, the high prevalence of bullying of children and youth with ASD (recently estimated at 46% of adolescents [50]) has made this form of victimization a critical consideration in educational contexts for those with ASD and their peers [51]. Specific effectiveness of mainstream bullying prevention programs for youth with ASD is unknown [50]; some have argued that bullying prevention and monitoring strategies should be part of the student's IEP, as well as a school-wide effort [52].

Post-secondary education

Educational opportunities and supports for older adolescents and young adults have come to the fore in recent years, as increasing numbers of more able individuals with ASD graduate from secondary schools. As yet, there is little evidence to support specific educational practices in this age range. However, the literature concerning other developmental and learning disorders provides some direction. Key factors include early assessment and preparation for realistic post-secondary options for the individual. Transition planning ideally begins in early adolescence and includes teaching skills related to self-determination (defined as the accumulation of skills, attitudes and beliefs enabling control over one's own life) as part of the educational curriculum (Table 6.4) [53]. Teaching such skills may be particularly essential yet uniquely challenging for individuals with ASD, for whom both sense of identity and ability to self-evaluate may be reduced relative to their peers [54], yet guidance from the literature is scarce.

- Educational programs must be individualized, based on profiles of strengths as well as weaknesses.
- Both academic and non-academic (eg, social, adaptive behavior) goals should be part of the individual plan, as appropriate.
- The future usefulness of any given skill to that individual should be taken into account before it becomes part of the teaching plan.
- Vigilance on the part of educators, parents and others is essential to prevent or address potential bullying/victimization.
- Formal planning for educational transitions (to middle or junior high school, to high school, to adulthood) should begin well in advance of the anticipated transition.

Table 6.4 Key considerations for educational programs for children with autism spectrum disorder.

Intervention for adults

Despite advances in intervention for younger individuals with ASD, data on outcomes in adulthood remain sobering. A recent epidemiological study in the UK showed that adults with ASD experienced high levels of unemployment and other economic disadvantages, as well as low levels of social support [55]. Reviews of research pertaining to services for adults with ASD highlight the anticipated increase in the already high need for services, accompanied by serious gaps in knowledge of effective practices [56,57]. As at all stages of the lifespan, the needs of adults with ASD vary enormously depending on level of function and presence of comorbid conditions [58]. Even among the most intellectually able persons with ASD, continuing supports are typically needed in work or other vocational settings. Thus, preparatory programs and supports are needed to enable participation in vocational activities (at whatever level meets individuals' abilities and interests), as are social skills programs and opportunities for social and community participation (Table 6.5).

• Given the limited research base, extrapolation from principles derived from interventions for younger individuals with autism spectrum disorder (ASD) is warranted.
• The need to respect adults' preferences regarding vocational activities and other life choices, and to ensure that programming is age-appropriate and contextually relevant, renders this period particularly sensitive for design and provision of intervention services.
• Access to mental health services is critical for adults with ASD.
• Support from individuals other than family members becomes an important consideration for addressing the long-term needs of adults with ASD. This issue is best addressed through early planning for transition to adulthood that recognizes the need to maximize independent living skills while family supports are still available.

Table 6.5 Key considerations for interventions for adults with autism spectrum disorder.

Appropriate residential options are also a critical issue for most adults with ASD, especially those with comorbid ID. A systematic review of psychosocial interventions for adults with ASD identified a range of single-case design studies of ABA-based interventions, and a few studies aimed at improving aspects of social cognition, as well as evaluations of a variety of community-based programs [59]. Overall, the evidence-base is limited and the majority of studies lack rigor. However, when there is a need to teach specific skills, or to reduce problem behavior, in order to accomplish valued goals for adults with ASD, the same principles of teaching and learning as described earlier for younger individuals apply equally to adults.

Treatment for associated mental health problems such as anxiety or depression is among the greatest areas of need for adults with ASD (see Chapter 3). Mental health services are also essential for adults with comorbid ID, who may present with aggressive behavior. Access to mental health practitioners with expertise in adapting psychotherapeutic approaches to the needs of clients with ASD is improving in major centers but remains a challenge in many areas. Experts highlight that the lack of coordination of the various services needed by most adults with ASD (eg, vocational, residential, recreational, mental health) is yet another service gap [57]. This challenge has been addressed for some adults with

ASD and ID in the context of community, residential, and vocational settings such as the Carolina Living and Learning Center, part of the statewide TEACCH system [60].

References

1 National Autism Center. National Standards Project. *Findings and conclusions addressing the need for evidence-based practice guidelines for autism spectrum disorders*. Randolph, MA: National Autism Center; 2009.

2 Cooper JO, Heron TE, Heward WL. *Applied Behavior Analysis*. Columbus, OH: Merrill; 2007.

3 Wong C, Odom SL, Hume K, et al. Evidence-based practices for children, youth, and young adults with Autism Spectrum Disorder. Chapel Hill: The University of North Carolina, Frank Porter Graham Child Development Institute, Autism Evidence-Based Practice Review Group. http://autismpdc.fpg.unc.edu/sites/autismpdc.fpg.unc.edu/files/2014-EBP-Report.pdf. Accessed February 4, 2015

4 Gast DL, Ledford JR, eds. *Single Subject Research Methodology in Behavioral Sciences*. New York, NY: Routledge; 2010.

5 Lovaas OI, Smith T. Early and intensive behavioral intervention in autism. In, Kazdin AE, and Weisz JR, eds. *Evidence-based Psychotherapies for Children and Adolescents*. New York, NY: Guilford Press; 2003:325-357.

6 Reichow B, Wolery M. Comprehensive synthesis of early intensive behavioral interventions for young children with autism based on the UCLA young autism project model. *J Autism Dev Disord.* 2009;39:23-41.

7 Reichow B. Overview of meta-analyses on early intensive behavioral intervention for young children with autism spectrum disorders. *J Autism Dev Disord*. 2012;42:512-520.

8 Reichow B, Barton EE, Boyd, BA, Hume, K. Early intensive behavioral intervention (EIBI) for young children with autism spectrum disorders (ASD). *Cochrane Database Syst Rev*. 2012; 10:CD009260.

9 Sallows GO, Graupner TD. Intensive behavioral treatment for children with autism: four-year outcome and predictors. *American J Mental Retardation*. 2005;110:417-438.

10 Flanagan HE, Perry A, Freeman NL. Effectiveness of a large-scale community-based Intensive Behavioral Intervention: A waitlist comparison study exploring outcomes and predictors. *Res Autism Spectr Disord*. 2012;6:673-682.

11 Perry A, Cummings A., Dunn Geier J, et al. Effectiveness of intensive behavioral intervention in a large, community-based program. *Res Autism Spectr Disord*. 2008;2:621-642.

12 Perry A, Cummings A., Dunn Geier, J et al. Predictors of outcome for children receiving intensive behavioral intervention in a large, community-based program. *Res Autism Spectr Disord*. 2011;5:592-603.

13 Smith IM, Koegel RL, Koegel LK, Openden DA, Fossum KL, Bryson SE. Effectiveness of a novel community-based early intervention model for children with autistic spectrum disorder. *Am J Intellect Dev Disabil*. 2010;115:504-523.

14 Fernell A, Hedvall A, Westerlund J, et al. Early intervention in 208 Swedish preschoolers with autism spectrum disorder. A prospective naturalistic study. *Res Dev Disabil.* 2011;32:2092-2101.

15 Boyd BA, Hume K, McBee MT, et al. Comparative efficacy of LEAP, TEACCH and non-model-specific special education programs for preschoolers with autism spectrum disorders. *J Autism Dev Disord.* 2014;44:366-380.

16 Dawson G, Rogers SJ, Munson J, et al. Randomized, controlled trial of an intervention for toddlers with autism: The Early Start Denver Model. *Pediatrics*. 2010;125:e17-e23.

17 Rogers SJ, Dawson G. *Early Start Denver Model for Young Children with Autism: Promoting Language, Learning, and Engagement*. New York, NY: Guilford Press; 2010.

18 National Research Council. Educating children with autism. In, Lord C, McGee JP, eds. *Committee on Educational Interventions for Children with Autism*. Washington DC: National Academy Press; 2001.

19 Keenan M, Kerr, KP, Dillenburger K. *Parents' Education as Autism Therapists*. London, UK: Jessica Kingsley; 2000.

20 Koegel LK, Koegel RL, Harrower JK, Carter CM. Pivotal response intervention I: Overview of approach. *J Assoc Pers Sev Handicaps*. 1999;24:174-185.

21 Koegel RL, Koegel LK. *Pivotal Response Treatments for Autism: Communication, Social, and Academic Development*. Baltimore, Maryland: Paul H. Brookes; 2006.

22 Stahmer AC, Gist K. The effects of an accelerated parent education program on technique mastery and child outcome. *J of Positive Behavior Interventions*. 2001;3:75-82.

23 Koegel RL, Koegel LK, O'Neill R. Generalization in the treatment of autism. In: McReynolds LV, Spradlin JE, eds. *Generalization Strategies in the Treatment of Communication Disorders*. Toronto, Canada: B.C. Decker; 1989:116-131

24 Minjarez MB, Williams SE, Mercier EM, Hardan AY. Pivotal response group treatment program for parents of children with autism. *J Autism Dev Disord*. 2011;41:92-101.

25 Coolican J, Smith IM, Bryson SE. Brief parent training in pivotal response treatment for preschoolers with autism. *J Child Psychol Psychiatry*. 2010;51:1321-1330.

26 Oono IP, Honey EJ, McConachie H. Parent-mediated early intervention for young children with autism spectrum disorders (ASD). *Cochrane Database Syst Rev*. 2013;4:CD009774.

27 Carter AS, Messinger DS, Stone WL, Celimli S, Nahmias AS, Yoder P. A randomized controlled trial of Hanen's 'More Than Words' in toddlers with early autism symptoms. *J Child Psychol Psychiatry*. 2011;52:741-752.

28 Green J, Charman T, McConachie H, et al; for the PACT Consortium. Parent-mediated communication-focused treatment in children with autism (PACT): a randomised controlled trial. *Lancet*. 2010;375:2152-2160.

29 Brookman-Frazee L, Vismara L, Drahota A, Stahmer A, Openden D. Parent training interventions for children with autism spectrum disorders. In, Matson JL, ed. *Applied Behavior Analysis for Children with Autism Spectrum Disorders*. New York, NY: Springer; 2009:237-257.

30 Patterson SY, Smith V, Mirenda P. A systematic review of training programs for parents of children with autism spectrum disorders: Single-subject contributions. *Autism*. 2012;16:498-522.

31 Schultz T, Schmidt C, Stichter JP. A review of parent education programs for parents of children with autism spectrum disorders. *Focus Autism Other Dev Disabil*. 2011;26:96-104.

32 Johnson CR, Handen BL, Butter E, et al. Develoment of a parent training program for children with pervasive developmental disorders. *Behav Interv*. 2007;22:201-221.

33 Scahill L, McDougle CJ, Aman MG, et al. Effects of risperidone and parent training on adaptive functioning in children with pervasive developmental disorders and serious behavioral problems: Research units on pediatric psychopharmacology autism network. *J Am Acad Child Adolesc Psychiatry*. 2012;51:136-146.

34 Carr EG, Dunlap G, Horner RH, et al. Positive Behavior Support: Evolution of an applied science. *J Posit Behav Interv*. 2002;4:4-16.

35 O'Neil RE, Horner RH, Albin, RW, Spragu J, Storey K, Newton JS, eds. *Functional Assessment and Program Development for Problem Behavior: A Practical Handbook*. 3rd edn. Stamford, CT: Cengage Learning; 2014.

36 Reichow B, Steiner AM, Volkmar F. Social skills groups for people aged 6 to 21 with autism spectrum disorders (ASD). *Cochrane Database Syst Rev*. 2012;7:CD00851.

37 Wang S, Parrila R, Cui Y. Meta-analysis of social skills interventions of single-case research for individuals with autism spectrum disorders: Results from three-level HLM. *J Autism Dev Disord*. 2013;43:1701-1716.

38 Mandelberg J, Laugeson EA, Cunningham TD, Ellingsen R, Bates S, Frankel F. Long-term treatment outcomes for parent-assisted social skills training for adolescents with autism spectrum disorders: The UCLA PEERS program. *J Ment Health Res Intellect Disabil*. 2014;7:45-73.

39 Laugeson EA, Frankel F, Gantam A, Dillon AR, Mogil C. Evidence-based social skills training for adolescents with autism spectrum disorders: the UCLA PEERS program. *J Autism Dev Disord*. 2012;42:1025-1036

40 Gantman A, Kapp SK, Orenski K, Laugeson EA. Social skills training for young adults with high-functioning autism spectrum disorders: a randomized controlled pilot study. *J Autism Dev Disord*. 2012;42:1094-1103.

41 Laugeson EA, Frankel F. *Social Skills for Teenagers with Developmental and Autism Spectrum Disorders: The PEERS Treatment Manual*. New York, NY: Routledge; 2010.

42 Laugeson EA. *The PEERS curriculum for School-Based Professionals: Social Skills Training for Adolescents with Autism Spectrum Disorder*. New York, NY: Routledge; 2014.

43 Zhang J, Wheeler JJ. A meta-analysis of peer-mediated interventions for young children with autism spectrum disorders. *Educ Train Autism Dev Disabil*. 2011;46:62-77.

44 Kasari C, Rotheram-Fuller E, Locke J, Gulsrud A. Making the connection: randomized controlled trial of social skills at school for children with autism spectrum disorders. *J Child Psychol Psychiatry*. 2012;53:431-439.

45 Klinger LG, O'Kelley SE, Mussey JL. Assessment of intellectual functioning in autism spectrum disorders. In, Goldstein S, Naglieri JA, Ozonoff S, eds. *Assessment of Autism Spectrum Disorders*. New York, NY: Guilford; 2009:209-252.

46 Corbett BA, Carmean V, Fein D. Assessment of neuropsychologicla functioning in autism spectrum disorders. In, Goldstein S, Naglieri JA, Ozonoff S, eds. *Assessment of Autism Spectrum Disorders*. New York, NY: Guilford; 2009:253-289.

47 Idring S, Rai D, Dal H, Dalman, C, Sturm H, et al. Autism spectrum disorders in the Stockholm Youth Cohort: Design, prevalence and validity. *PLoS ONE*. 2012:7:e41280.

48 American Psychiatric Association. *Diagnostic and Statistical Manual of Mental Disorders*. 5th edn. Arlington, VA: American Psychiatric Publishing; 2012.

49 National Autism Center (NAC). Evidence-based practice and autism in the schools. Randolph, MA: National Autism Center; 2009b. NAC website. www.nationalautismcenter.org/pdf/NAC%20Ed%20Manual_FINAL.pdf. Accessed February 4, 2015.

50 Sterzing PR, Shattuck PT, Narendorf SC, Wagner M, Cooper BP. Bullying involvement and autism spectrum disorders: prevalence and correlates of bullying involvement among adolescents with an autism spectrum disorder. *Arch Pediatr Adolesc Med*. 2012;166:1058-1064.

51 Hebron J, Humphrey N. Exposure to bullying among students with autism spectrum conditions: a multi-informant analysis of risk and protective factors. *Autism*. 2013; 18:618-630.

52 Cappadocia MC, Weiss JA, Pepler. Bullying experiences among children and youth with autism spectrum disorders. *J Autism Dev Disord*. 2012; 42:266-277.

53 Wehmeyer ML, Agran M, Hughes C, Martin JE, Mithaug DE, Palmer SB. Promoting self-determination in students with developmental disabilities. New York, NY: Guilford; 2007.

54 Johnson SA, Filliter JH, Murphy RR. Discrepancies between self- and parent-perceptions of autistic traits and empathy in high functioning children and adolescents on the autism spectrum. *J Autism Dev Disord*. 2009;39:1706-1714.

55 Brugha TS, McManus S, Bankart J, et al. The epidemiology of autism spectrum disorders in adults in the community in England. *Arch Gen Psychiatry*. 2011;68:459-466.

56 Howlin P, Moss P. Adults with autism spectrum disorders. *Can J Psychiatry*. 2012;57:275-283.

57 Shattuck PT, Roux AM, Hudson LE, Taylor JL, Maenner MJ, Trani JF. Services for adults with an autism spectrum disorder. *Can J Psychiatry*. 2012;57:284-291.

58 Taylor JL, Selzer MM. Changes in the autism behavioral phenotype during the transition to adulthood. *J Autism Dev Disord*. 2010;40:1431-1446.

59 Bishop-Fitzpatrick L, Minshew N, Eack S. A systematic review of psychosocial interventions for adults with autism spectrum disorders. *J Autism Dev Disord*. 2013;43:687-694.

60 Van Bourgondien ME, Reichle NC, Schopler E. Effects of a model treatment approach on adults with autism. *J Autism Dev Disord*. 2003;33:131-140.

Chapter 7

Autism spectrum disorder and the family: examining impacts and the need for support

David B Nicholas and Christopher Kilmer

Key Learning Objectives

By the end of this chapter, readers will be able to:

- understand psychosocial impacts of autism spectrum disorder (ASD) on individuals and families;
- understand ways that families navigate ASD-associated care;
- gain knowledge about family experiences in the context of transition and lifespan issues; and
- identify emerging questions and priorities for understanding family issues and supporting family wellness.

Introduction

ASD is a pervasive condition that has a profound and prolonged impact on families. This chapter offers an overview of selected literature identifying family experiences of ASD, with implications for clinical care and support. An argument is made for greater person- and family-centered care, including reflective practice that enables heightened understanding and support for families with the aim of optimal individual and family experience.

E. Anagnostou and J. Brian (eds.), *Clinician's Manual on Autism Spectrum Disorder*, DOI 10.1007/978-3-319-03056-2_7

Impact of autism spectrum disorder on families

ASD presents many challenges that can profoundly affect family life. The heterogeneity of ASD and the uniqueness of families cumulatively lead to a wide variety of experiences and outcomes. Outcomes are further affected by external factors and social determinants such as socioeconomic status, funding availability for services, geographic location and proximity to services, parental availability for family-mediated intervention, broader community support, and a range of other considerations.

Notwithstanding this variation of family experience, ASD invariably affects individuals within the family and the family as a whole. As an example, external factors such as funding limitations, lengthy waiting times, and strict eligibility requirements affect the roles that parents play in accessing and delivering interventions. In seeking services, parents typically assume roles of advocate and coordinator of their child's care, which imposes demands on parents and often relegates them to service access pathways that are rife with confusion, uncertainty, and stress [1–3].

Emerging evidence points to qualitative differences in parenting a child with ASD. Studies increasingly attest to nuanced tasks associated with parental care for a child with ASD, manifested as extraordinary work that can span day- and night-time hours, often leaving parents sleep-deprived and emotionally strained [4–6].

There are current gaps in our understanding about how families make meaning of ASD and integrate this specialized care within family life, as seen with recent efforts to address the critical role that parents play in the life of their child with ASD [4]. This work highlights a range of tensions experienced by parents. For instance, from the initial awareness of ASD-like symptoms in their child, parents describe difficulty obtaining a diagnosis for their child often due to long delays for a developmental assessment. Ironically, some of the strengths that parents may see in their child (eg, organization of items) are often recast at diagnosis as an illustration of differences associated with ASD. Parents' relentless need to advocate for services renders a complex conundrum and, in particular, a discourse that warrants early and substantial child intervention often in the face of restrictions and delays in obtaining funding and accessing services. Using the National Survey of Children With Special Health Care Needs, Kogan et al [7] compared groups of 3–17-year-old children with:

- special health care needs and ASD;
- special health care needs and other developmental, behavioral, or emotional challenges; and
- other special health care needs.

The group of parents whose child had special health care needs and ASD were more likely to report substantial financial costs, including a reduction of employment in order to care for their child [7]. A ten-year longitudinal ethnographic study exploring the psychosocial elements of parenting a child with ASD demonstrated that, while parents exhibited high levels of psychological distress, this lessened as the child advanced in age (although distress levels remained substantial) [8]. Career difficulties were also experienced, more typically by mothers than fathers. While some mothers had entered the workforce or were pursuing education, approximately half reported being either unable to work or requiring a restricted schedule or type of employment [8]. Parents were also found to be concerned about a loss of family opportunity to socialize due to having a child with ASD. Generally, and continuing over time, approximately 20% reported this as a problematic, long-standing issue.

Some problems faced by families, such as child communication and behavioral issues in public, were reported to diminish over time; however, in some cases, other problems developed or intensified over time, such as parental anxiety over their child's future or the possibility of increased aggressive behavior [8]. Hastings and colleagues explored the coping strategies of parents of children with ASD and found that mothers and fathers may cope differently [9]. Yet more research is warranted to address parental coping and differential impacts of ASD between mothers and fathers. While these differences are hypothesized, little research has yet examined potential differences.

Impact on parenting

Gray examined parental experience with a focus on the ongoing imposition of stigma [8]. This construct was further differentiated as 'felt' and 'enacted' stigma. The majority of parents of a child with ASD experienced both forms, with mothers being more likely than fathers to report stigma [8]. Felt stigma commonly occurred when in public settings. During these occasions, parents believed that others were judging their parenting abilities. Enacted stigma was less common, being reported by about half of the participants. It reflected forms of avoidance (eg, not being invited to social events), members of the public staring at the family in what was described as a 'hostile' manner, and individuals making rude or hurtful comments to members of the family. Parents reported heightened difficulties with stigma due to ASD not being a visible disability [8]. In another study, Gray reported that while social stigma was experienced by parents across the study's decade-long time frame, it mattered less to parents as time progressed [10].

Woodgate, Ateah, and Secco [5] interviewed parents of children with ASD about their experience and the main themes that emerged included:

- '*living in a world of our own*': feeling alone and isolated from peers, family, and society, and in many cases, not having an accessible support system of professionals;
- '*vigilant parenting*': extensive and protective practices that parents enacted, as well as viewing parenting as a team effort;
- '*sustaining the self and family*': belief that a strong sense of self and family and a healthy familial balance is beneficial to the child with ASD; and
- '*fighting all the way*': parents felt that they needed to assume an advocacy role for their family, as well as seek to improve the system for other families in which a child has ASD. Parent education was highlighted as important in navigating and managing ASD in daily life.

Bayat [11] explored the notion of resiliency among families in which a child has ASD. Based on survey results, family resiliency was identified as being present in families; however, this was manifested in a number of ways. For instance, participants reported their family pulling together and becoming more cohesive, finding meaning in the hardships they encountered, achieving increased personal strength and ability to be compassionate, and fostering a deeper sense of spirituality [11].

Impact on siblings

Macks and Reeve [12] explored the psychosocial and emotional adjustment of siblings of children with ASD by comparing this group to a comparison group of children whose sibling(s) did not have a disability. Interestingly, siblings of children with ASD had a more positive view of themselves relative to peers' self-appraisal regarding their behavior and intelligence [12]. However, certain demographic characteristics were more likely to negatively affect the sibling of a child with ASD, such as low socioeconomic status, being an only other sibling, and being older than the child with ASD. Benson and Karlof similarly examined the adjustment of siblings of a child with ASD compared to children without a sibling with ASD [13]. The level of parental involvement in education was related to positive sibling adjustment. Stressful life events, such as financial issues and the death of friends or family members, were reported to have an adverse effect on sibling adjustment. The quality of 'family climate' was linked with heightened prosocial behavior [13].

Impact on grandparents

Relatively little research has examined grandparenting in ASD. Margetts et al explored the experiences of grandparents of a child with ASD through qualitative interviews [14]. Grandparents reported a 'parental bond,' yet also described a burden of caring for both their grandchild with ASD and the grandchild's parent (ie, their adult child). Another emergent theme comprised grandparental 'striving for answers,' as grandparents struggled with how to best support their adult children and what role they should play, while at the same time attempting to understand ASD. 'Keeping intact,' the final theme presented by Margetts et al, entailed grandparental attempts to discover and establish their role within the family, with some grandparents feeling a responsibility to keep the family intact [14].

Navigating the transition to adulthood

As children with ASD advance toward adulthood, families are faced with additional challenges amidst a relative dearth of information or resources related to transitional and lifespan-based issues. Parents report varying needs related to mental health concerns such as anxiety and depression, sensory issues, vocation, housing, and other areas of concern. Resources for youth and adults are integral to establishing and enabling a viable life plan that optimizes opportunity and quality of life. Yet, parents often have no, few, and/or underdeveloped resources [15] and face a myriad of barriers to meaningful community engagement for their adult child. Service systems vary across jurisdiction but are generally insufficient to meet needs [16,17].

With multiple demands of care and a largely 'siloed' (ie, restricted to particular services) adult service system in regard to funding, health care, mental health, vocational training, and housing, parents are often left to independently struggle in seeking, finding, and coordinating services.

Considerations following a diagnosis of autism spectrum disorder

There is a current gap in our understanding about how families affected by ASD move forward and reconcile their lives relative to the presence of ASD. Little has been published on the cumulative impact of ASD on families over time. Questions abound such as:

- How do couples navigate and mutually manage ASD in the context of child and adolescent development?
- What is the impact of ASD on the parents' relationship as a couple (or other co-parenting partner configurations)?
- What strategies optimally support families as they navigate ASD care and manage family life?

While examples of excellent care exist, there is substantial work to be done in order to consistently offer effective supports for all families throughout the lifespan of the individual with ASD. Understanding the trajectory of the family requires increased family-based research. To that end, sensitive metrics are needed to understand and monitor the impact of ASD on the family and assess how ASD is understood and managed in daily life. For clinicians, assessment and support services need to more comprehensively consider the needs of the entire family. Thorough assessment, followed by corresponding resources, would result in greater understanding, improved outcomes, and better-supported families.

Finally, theoretically-grounded models need to be developed that fully recognize and value the role of the family in care provision and outcomes. Existing examples include the Bowen Theory, a family systems approach which accounts for the interaction of subsystems and recognizes how one member of the family influences another [18]; however, how a person with ASD uniquely nuances this process is still largely unknown. Further development and refinement of this and similar models may support our quest to more fully understand how ASD affects family life and how family functioning moderates the impact of ASD. Moreover, critically considering and redressing structural and community barriers associated with the social determinants of health can assist in mitigating inequities faced by marginalized families in contemporary society.

Implications for practitioners

There is a pressing need to achieve better outcomes for families affected by ASD. Advancement seems to entail increased investment in clinical and community care, research, and education, with an aim of evidence-based models of practice and capacity development. In advocating for this advancement, several considerations emerge.

First, many individuals with ASD experience comorbid health, mental health, and sensory issues. Given the preponderance and complexity of these challenges in the lives of individuals with ASD and their families, there is a need for timely assessment and proactive follow-up in effectively responding to these comorbidities (see Chapters 3 and 4). Proactive intervention is not only important for the individual with ASD but also her/his family, which often buffers the challenges associated with these issues. Practitioners need to carefully examine the extent to which clinical, educational, vocational, and other community environments impose conditions that heighten anxiety or discomfort for the individual with ASD. Strategies to neutralize stress-inducing environments or conditions warrant strategic planning and management. This may include new models advancing comprehensive and coordinated care in the community.

Families have presented a range of positive and negative experiences with ASD service providers and systems [4]. Emerging evidence highlights the promising effect of child and family-centered care in nurturing constructive experiences and satisfaction for families [19]. Person- and family-centered care offer an integral component to pediatric and adult care; these principles inviting professional reflection on ways to foster respect, information sharing and collaboration with families [20].

Consistent with person- and family-centered care, service providers are well-advised to listen to parents who tend to be knowledgeable advocates for their loved one with ASD. Parental perspectives can be pivotal to the acquisition of case-related knowledge and astute planning. This is particularly salient if the person with ASD is non-verbal or has a cognitive impairment that precludes independent communication of personal needs and wants.

Thus, training at multiple levels in ASD to complement person- and family-centered care, is recommended. Infusing ASD and family-centered curricula in to trainee education and professional development can increase practitioner capacity. A multipronged capacity-building approach is sought that includes learning opportunities for individuals with ASD, parents, families, lay supporters, and communities, as well as interdisciplinary education for community practitioners, medical subspecialists, and allied health care professionals caring for related health and mental health issues (eg, gastrointestinal issues, seizures, psychiatric concerns).

Conclusions

Understanding the strengths and challenges of individuals and families living with ASD is critically important, as is supporting families with proactive strategies via accessible and evidence-informed person- and family-centered care. This invites a comprehensive and coordinated care system with defined targets. Clearly, much work has yet to be done, but steps forward include greater awareness of families' experiences, priorities, and needs, and the corresponding development of adequately funded resources for individuals and families. Intentionally partnering with families can take us a long way towards building impactful relationships of engagement and support.

References

1 Kabot S, Masi W, Segal M. Advances in the diagnosis and treatment of autism spectrum disorders. *Prof Psychol Res Pr.* 2003;34:26-33.

2 Marcus LM, Kunce LJ, Schopler E. Working with Families. In, Cohen DJ, Volkmar FR, eds. *Handbook of Autism and Pervasive Developmental Disorders.* 2nd edn. New York: John Wiley and Sons; 1997:631-649.

3 Stoddart KP. *Reported stress, personality, and mental health in parents of children with pervasive developmental disorders.* Faculty of Social Work, University of Toronto, Toronto; 2003.

4 Nicholas DB, Zwaigenbaum L, Roberts W, McKeever P. Examining the experience of mothers of children with autism. Canadian Paediatric Society 90th Annual Conference. Edmonton, Canada. June 19-21, 2013.

5 Woodgate RL, Ateah C, Secco L. Living in a world of our own: The experience of parents who have a child with autism. *Qual Health Res.* 2008;18:1075-1083.

6 Lutz HR, Patterson BJ, Klein J. Coping with autism: A journey toward adaptation. *J Pediatr Nurs.* 2012;27:206-213.

7 Kogan MD, Strickland BB, Blumberg SJ, Singh GK, Perrin JM, van Dyck PC. A national profile of health care experiences and family impact of autism spectrum disorder among children in the United States, 2005-2006. *Pediatrics.* 2008;122:e1149-e1158.

8 Gray DE. 'Everybody just freezes. Everybody is just embarrassed': Felt and enacted stigma among parents of children with high functioning autism. *Sociol Health Illn.* 2002a;24:734-749.

9 Hastings RP, Kovshoff H, Brown T, Ward NJ, Espinosa FD, Remington B. Coping strategies in mothers and fathers of preschool and school-age children with autism. *Autism.* 2005;9:377-391.

10 Gray DE. Ten years on: A longitudinal study of families of children with autism. *J Intellect Dev Disabil.* 2002b;27:215-222.

11 Bayat M. Evidence of resilience in families of children with autism. *J Intellect Dev Disabil.* 2007;51:702-714.

12 Macks RJ, Reeve RE. The adjustment of non-disabled siblings of children with autism. *J Autism Dev Disord.* 2007;37:1060-1067.

13 Benson PR, Karlof KL. Child, parent, and family predictors of latter adjustment in siblings of children with autism. *Res Autism Spectr Disord.* 2008;2:583-600.

14 Margetts JK, Le Couteur A, Croom S. Families in a state of flux: The experiences of grandparents in autism spectrum disorder. *Child Care Health Dev.* 2006;32:565-574.

15 Nicholas DB, Attridge M, Zwaigenbaum L, Clarke M. Vocational support approaches in autism spectrum disorder: a synthesis review of the literature. *Autism.* 2014;19:235-245.

16 World Health Organization. Autism spectrum disorders and other developmental disorders: From raising awareness to building capacity. www.who.int/mental_health/maternal-child/autism_report/en/. WHO website. Updated 2013. Accessed February 4, 2015.

17 The Standing Senate Committee on Social Affairs, Science and Technology. Pay now or pay later: Autism families in crisis. www.parl.gc.ca/Content/SEN/Committee/391/soci/rep/repfinmar07-e.htm. Updated March 2007. Accessed February 4, 2015.

18 Bowen Center for the Family. The Bowen theory. www.thebowencenter.org/pages/theory.html. Accessed February 4, 2015.

19 Nicholas DB, Keilty K, Karmali K. Paediatric patient-centred care: Evidence and evolution. In, Zlotnik Shaul R, ed. *Ethics and Law in Pediatric Patient and Family-Centred Care.* New York, NY: Springer; 2014.

20 Institute for Patient- and Family-Centered Care (IPFCC). Frequently Asked Questions. IPFCC website. www.ipfcc.org/faq.html. Accessed February 4, 2015.

Chapter 8

Future directions

Jessica Brian, Evdokia Anagnostou

With rising prevalence rates, improvements in early detection, and increased awareness overall, autism spectrum disorder (ASD) will increasingly be in the purview of primary care physicians and other community practitioners. In light of these developments, primary care providers will benefit from arming themselves with knowledge about the state of the science in ASD and best practices for care. We now understand ASD to have a strong genomic/epigenomic contribution and we have an accumulation of evidence to inform earliest detection, timely diagnosis, and behavioral interventions. Primary care providers are tasked with understanding the most common co-occurring medical and psychiatric/mental health conditions in individuals with ASD, and will increasingly find themselves in a position to counsel and support individuals and their families, and to treat these co-occurring conditions. By adopting a person- and family-centred approach, care providers will be able to appreciate the unique stressors and joys associated with raising a child with ASD and will be better able to support not only the families, but the individuals themselves as they develop through the lifespan. While there remain many instances where specialists and/or specialized teams will be needed, we increasingly recognize the essential role of primary care providers in contributing to the well-being of individuals with ASD and their families.

E. Anagnostou and J. Brian (eds.), *Clinician's Manual on Autism Spectrum Disorder*, DOI 10.1007/978-3-319-03056-2_8

Future advances

As we look ahead into the next generation(s), advances in several key areas will have a major impact on the ASD experience for individuals and families. These, in turn, will affect how we provide care and counsel patients. Significant advances are on the horizon in:

- genomics/epigenomics;
- detection of very early behavioral markers;
- characterization of comborbidities;
- psychopharmacological treatments;
- behavioral interventions; and
- person- and family-centered care.

Advances in genomics/epigenomics

Significant advances have been made in recent years in our understanding of the genomic contribution to ASD. We know that first-degree relatives of children with ASD are at increased risk for ASD and related outcomes themselves [1]. However, most genomic variation discovered to date in ASD is still de novo, and evidence supports a major role of epigenomics in the expression of ASD [2]. The more we learn about genomic variation, the closer we will come to being able to map down to metabolic pathways, which will inform the identification of biological subgroups. This in turn will inform the development of targeted treatments.

Advances in early detection

The average age of diagnosis remains around 4 years of age in most industrialized nations despite impressive advances in early detection research (eg, Autism Speaks' Baby Siblings Research Consortium, which includes research teams from Canada, Israel, the United Kingdom, and the United States). A host of early risk markers have been identified as early as 12 months of age in high-risk babies (ie, siblings of children with ASD, who themselves are at increased risk), suggesting that the age of detection could be significantly younger [1,3]. Earlier detection is a priority given evidence of improved outcomes with earlier intervention [4]. This is supported by current understanding of neural plasticity which would predict the mitigation of downstream effects of biological atypicalities in response to earlier intervention. In order to move this work forward, we will need to determine the predictive value of these risk markers in other at-risk and typically developing populations (eg, to establish their specificity to ASD or related suboptimal outcomes), disseminate this evidence effectively to community practitioners, provide training opportunities in the assessment and detection of these early signs, and promote models of service delivery that support earlier identification and diagnosis. Such advances have the potential to substantially improve timely access to appropriate care at the earliest time points, thus increasing the potential for optimal outcomes.

Exploring comorbidities

Both medical and psychiatric comorbidities are common in ASD. There is still a lot of work to be done to understand whether the constructs of these comorbidities are the same in patients with ASD as in the general population (eg, is anxiety in ASD the same disorder as anxiety in the general population? Are gastointestinal issues in ASD simply co-occurring or linked to the pathophysiology of the disorder?). Stratification by medical and/or psychiatric comorbidities will contribute to the success of clinical trials research.

Developments in psychopharmacological treatments

New molecular and circuitry targets are emerging from genomics, neuropathology, and systems neuroscience. The task now is to start translating such findings into treatments that specifically address the pathophysiology of differences in ASD. Emerging biomarker discovery will also become critical to allow for personalization of treatments based on individual biological and other differences.

Future developments in behavioral intervention research

Prior to recent years, the majority of evidence supporting behavioral intervention had come from single-subject designs and smaller studies from highly specialized academic centers. Only very recently has there been a ground swell of evidence from larger-scale investigations, including randomized controlled trials, meta-analyses, and wide-scale community dissemination studies. Next steps for behavioral intervention efforts, already emerging, include addressing the developmental needs of babies/toddlers in the first years of life [5], the development and evaluation of interventions based on emerging signs of risk (rather than waiting for confirmed diagnosis), the greater inclusion of primary caregivers (parents, grandparents, childcare providers), and models that increase timely access to care by improving feasibility, cost-effectiveness, portability, and ease of community implementation.

Advances in person- and family-centered care

Recent developments include the increased appreciation of the family's role in the lives of children with ASD, with the promise of ongoing investigation of caregiver burden, identification of needs during transitions throughout the lifespan, and the lived experience of individuals with ASD and their family members. Many questions remain about the impact of ASD on the family as a unit, on the parents' relationship with one another, and on individual family members, but this important area of research is gaining traction and is increasingly recognized as a research priority.

Conclusions

As the need for ASD care has increased, so has the appreciation of the complexity inherent in this multifactorial disorder. Heterogeneity exists in the underlying biology, etiology, developmental progression, behavioral presentation, individual and family experience, associated medical and psychiatric conditions, and not surprisingly, in the response to intervention for individuals with ASD. This complexity presents unique challenges to individuals and their families, researchers, care providers, and policy-makers. By working together to further propel research efforts and improve access to timely, high quality care, we will enter the next decade armed with the tools to reduce the burden and optimize outcomes for individuals with ASD and their caregivers.

References

1 Ozonoff S, Young GS, Carter A, et al. Recurrence risk for autism spectrum disorders: a Baby Siblings Research Consortium study. *Pediatrics*. 2011;128:e488-e495.

2 Anagnostou E, Zwaigenbaum L, Szatmari P, et al. Autism spectrum disorder: advances in evidence-based practice. *CMAJ*. 2014;186:509-519.

3 Zwaigenbaum L, Bryson S, Lord C, et al. Clinical assessment and management of toddlers with suspected autism spectrum disorder: insights from studies of high-risk infants. *Pediatrics*. 2009;123:1383-1391.

4 Makrygianni MK, Reed P. A meta-analytic review of the effectiveness of behavioural early intervention programs for children with Autistic Spectrum Disorders. *Res Autism Spectr Disord*. 2010;4:577-593.

5 Brian JA, Bryson SE, Zwaigenbaum L. Autism spectrum disorder in infancy: developmental considerations in treatment targets. *Current Opin Neurol*. 2015; 28:117-123.

MIX
Papier aus verantwortungsvollen Quellen
Paper from responsible sources
FSC® C105338

If you have any concerns about our products,
you can contact us on
ProductSafety@springernature.com

In case Publisher is established outside the EU,
the EU authorized representative is:
Springer Nature Customer Service Center GmbH
Europaplatz 3, 69115 Heidelberg, Germany

Printed by Libri Plureos GmbH
in Hamburg, Germany